T0259315

Clinical Applications of Probiotics in Gastroenterology: Questions and Answers

Editor

GERALD FRIEDMAN

GASTROENTEROLOGY CLINICS OF NORTH AMERICA

www.gastro.theclinics.com

December 2012 • Volume 41 • Number 4

ELSEVIER

Elsevier Inc. • 1600 John F. Kennedy Blvd., Suite 1800 • Philadelphia, Pennsylvania 19103-2899
http://www.theclinics.com

GASTROENTEROLOGY CLINICS OF NORTH AMERICA Volume 41, Number 4
December 2012 ISSN 0889-8553, ISBN-13: 978-1-4557-4913-3

Editor: Kerry Holland
Developmental Editor: Donald Mumford

Gastroenterology Clinics of North America (ISSN 0889-8553) is published quarterly by Elsevier Inc., 360 Park Avenue South, New York, NY 10010-1710. Months of issue are March, June, September, and December. Business and Editorial Offices: 1600 John F. Kennedy Blvd., Suite 1800, Philadelphia, PA 19103-2899. Customer Service Office: 6277 Sea Harbor Drive, Orlando, FL 32887-4800. Periodicals postage paid at New York, NY and additional mailing offices. Subscription prices are $305.00 per year (US individuals), $153.00 per year (US students), $488.00 per year (US institutions), $335.00 per year (Canadian individuals), $594.00 per year (Canadian institutions), $423.00 per year (international individuals), $211.00 per year (international students), and $594.00 per year (international institutions). Foreign air speed delivery is included in all *Clinics* subscription prices. All prices are subject to change without notice. **POSTMASTER**: Send address changes to *Gastroenterology Clinics of North America*, Elsevier Health Sciences Division, Subscription Customer Service, 3251 Riverport Lane, Maryland Heights, MO 63043. Telephone: 1-800-654-2452 (U.S. and Canada); 314-447-8871 (outside U.S. and Canada). Fax: 314-447-8029. E-mail: journalscustomerservice-usa@elsevier.com (for print support); journalsonlinesupport-usa@elsevier.com (for online support).

Reprints. For copies of 100 or more, of articles in this publication, please contact the Commercial Reprints Department, Elsevier Inc., 360 Part Avenue South, New York, New York 10010-1710. Tel. (212) 633-3813, Fax: (212) 462-1935, E-mail: reprints@elsevier.com.

Gastroenterology Clinics of North America is also published in Italian by Il Pensiero Scientifico Editore, Rome, Italy; and in Portuguese by Interlivros Edicoes Ltda., Rua Commandante Coelho 1085, 21250 Cordovil, Rio de Janeiro, Brazil.

Gastroenterology Clinics of North America is covered in *MEDLINE/PubMed (Index Medicus)*, *Excerpta Medica*, *Current Contents/Clinical Medicine*, *Science Citation Index*, *ISI/BIOMED*, and *BIOSIS*.

Printed and bound by CPI Group (UK) Ltd, Croydon, CR0 4YY

Transferred to digital print 2012

Contributors

GUEST EDITOR

GERALD FRIEDMAN, MD, PhD, MS, FACP, MACG, AGAF
Clinical Professor of Medicine, The Mount Sinai School of Medicine, New York, New York

AUTHORS

THOMAS JULIUS BORODY, MD, PhD
Director, Centre for Digestive Diseases, Five Dock, New South Wales, Australia

JORDANA CAMPBELL, BSc
Research Officer, Centre for Digestive Diseases, Five Dock, New South Wales, Australia

MAURIZIO CASSADER, PhD
Department of Medical Sciences, University of Turin, Turin, Italy

ANNE M. DATTILO, PhD, RD
Nestlé Nutrition, Medical Scientific and Regulatory Unit, Florham Park, New Jersey

DENNY DEMERIA, MD, FRCPC
Gastroenterologist, Division of Gastroenterology, University of Alberta, Edmonton, Alberta, Canada

RICHARD FEDORAK, MD, FRCP, FRCP(London), FRS
Professor of Medicine, Division of Gastroenterology, University of Alberta, Edmonton, Alberta, Canada

GERALD FRIEDMAN, MD, PhD, MS, FACP, MACG, AGAF
Clinical Professor of Medicine, Mount Sinai School of Medicine, New York, New York

ROBERTO GAMBINO, PhD
Department of Medical Sciences, University of Turin, Turin, Italy

KRISTON GANGULI, MD
Instructor in Pediatrics, Mucosal Immunology Laboratory, Division of Pediatric Gastroenterology, Massachusetts General Hospital for Children, Harvard Medical School, Charlestown, Massachusetts

ERIKA ISOLAURI, MD, PhD
Professor, Department of Paediatrics, University of Turku and Turku University Hospital, Turku, Finland

BLAIR LAWLEY, PhD
Department of Microbiology and Immunology, University of Otago, Dunedin, New Zealand

FEDERICA MOLINARO, MD
Department of Medical Sciences, University of Turin, Turin, Italy

GIOVANNI MUSSO, MD
Department of Emergency Medicine, Gradenigo Hospital, Gradenigo Hospital, Turin, Italy

ELENA PASCHETTA, MD
Department of Medical Sciences, University of Turin, Turin, Italy

EAMONN M.M. QUIGLEY, MD, FRCP, FACP, FACG, FRCPI
Professor of Medicine and Human Physiology, Department of Medicine, Alimentary Pharmabiotic Centre, University College Cork, Cork, Ireland

SAMULI RAUTAVA, MD, PhD
Department of Paediatrics, University of Turku and Turku University Hospital, Turku, Finland

JOSÉ M. SAAVEDRA, MD
Department of Pediatrics, Johns Hopkins University School of Medicine, Baltimore, Maryland; Nestlé Nutrition, Medical Scientific and Regulatory Unit, Florham Park, New Jersey

SEPPO SALMINEN, PhD
Professor, Functional Foods Forum, University of Turku, Turku, Finland

FERGUS SHANAHAN, MD
Professor and Chair, Department of Medicine, Alimentary Pharmabiotic Centre, University College Cork, National University of Ireland, Cork, Ireland

GERALD W. TANNOCK, PhD
Department of Microbiology and Immunology, University of Otago, Dunedin, New Zealand; Riddet Institute Centre of Research Excellence, Massey University, Palmerston North, New Zealand

W. ALLAN WALKER, MD
Professor in Pediatrics, Mucosal Immunology Laboratory, Division of Pediatric Gastroenterology, Massachusetts General Hospital for Children, Harvard Medical School, Charlestown, Massachusetts

Contents

> Gut microbiota constitute a highly complex ecosystem that interacts with the host and profoundly affects gastrointestinal and systemic immunologic functions. Specific microbial patterns are associated with healthy children and adults, and these patterns are greatly related to the early acquisition of microbes by the newborn and the development of gut microbial communities in the perinatal period. Although direct causation must be firmly established and mechanisms fully elucidated, strong and increasing evidence shows that the early acquisition, development, and maintenance of specific bacterial populations are critical to human health, and a better understanding of these offers great opportunities for intervention.

> Necrotizing enterocolitis (NEC) is a devastating condition characterized by diffuse intestinal inflammation and necrosis in preterm infants. It is the most common gastrointestinal emergency in the neonatal intensive care unit and is associated with significant morbidity and mortality. Primary risk factors include prematurity and low birth weight. Although the pathogenesis of NEC is complex and not entirely understood, it is known that an interplay between immature intestinal immune responses and the process of bacterial colonization is required for the development of this disease.

> Gut microbiota composition can discriminate between allergic and healthy children, and the distinction may precede clinical manifestations of disease. The mother provides the first inoculum of bacteria, which influences the risk of becoming allergic later in life. Bifidobacterium species are major determinants of disease risk. Specific probiotics may modulate early microbial colonization, which represents the first intervention target in allergic disease, together with their ability to reverse the increased intestinal permeability characteristic of children with atopic eczema and food allergy. Probiotics also enhance gut-specific IgA responses, which are frequently defective in children with food allergy. In addition, probiotics have the potential to alleviate allergic inflammation locally and systemically.

Obesity-related disorders derive from a combination of genetic suscepti-bility and environmental factors. Recent evidence supports the role of gut microbiota in the pathogenesis of obesity, type 2 diabetes mellitus, and insulin resistance by increasing energy harvest from diet and by induc-ing chronic, low-grade inflammation. Several studies describe characteris-tic differences between composition and activity of gut microbiota of lean individuals and those with obesity. Despite this evidence, some patho-physiological mechanisms remain to be clarified. This article discusses mechanisms connecting gut microbiota to obesity and fat storage and the potential therapeutic role of probiotics and prebiotics.

This article describes nucleic acid-based methods to assess the compo-sition and function of the bowel microbiota. The methods range from the relatively simple (polymerase chain reaction) to the technically sophisti-cated (metatranscriptomics). Not all are accessible to the majority of lab-oratories, but a core of validated (used in more than 1 study) tools is readily available to most researchers. Reliance on a single methodology per human study is not recommended. Generally, a study could com-mence with a screening of samples to determine whether it will be worth-while expending further time and money on an in-depth analysis.

Probiotics have a long record of safety, which relates primarily to lactoba-cilli and bifidobacteria. Experience with other forms of probiotic is more limited. There is no such thing as zero risk, particularly in the context of certain forms of host susceptibility. There is poor public understanding of the concept of risk, in general, and risk/benefit analysis, in particular. Uncertainty persists regarding the potential for transfer of antibiotic resis-tance with probiotics, but the risk seems to be low with currently available probiotic products. As with other forms of therapeutics, the safety of pro-biotics should be considered on a strain-by-strain basis.

GASTROENTEROLOGY
CLINICS OF NORTH AMERICA

DOWNLOAD
Free App!

Review Articles
THE CLINICS

NOW AVAILABLE FOR YOUR iPhone and iPad

Preface

Clinical Applications of Probiotics in Gastroenterology: Questions and Answers

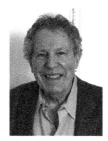

Gerald Friedman, MD, PhD, MS, FACP, MACG, AGAF
Guest Editor

Seven years have passed since the publication of "Probiotics, Prebiotics, and Commensal Bacteria: Perspectives and Clinical Applications in Gastroenterology" appeared in *Gastroenterology Clinics of North America* (2005). Since that time a vast amount of knowledge related to commensal bacteria and probiotics has been accumulated through the work of basic scientists and clinicians. The Microbiome Project commenced in 2007 and contributions worldwide have intensified the quest for knowledge regarding the role of commensal bacteria in the genesis of the immune system as well as the role of intestinal microbiota in health and disease. This issue represents a select group of outstanding national and international investigators and clinicians who provide extensive expertise and insight related to the practical applications of probiotics in a variety of clinical settings.

Dr Molinaro and associates note that obesity-related disorders are associated with energy homeostasis and inflammation. Gut microbiota are involved in several host metabolic functions and may play an important role by increasing energy harvest from the diet, by regulating host metabolism, and by modulating inflammation. Experimental data suggest that manipulation of gut microbiota with prebiotics and probiotics can beneficially transiently affect adiposity and glucose metabolism. The authors analyze the potential gut microbiota–driven pathways that could represent novel targets for the treatment of obesity.

Drs Saavedra and Dattilo provide significant information regarding the role of early acquisition of microbiota in the perinatal period and the development of immune function. The time of development, the microbial profile, and the diversity of this ecosystem

Gastroenterol Clin N Am 41 (2012) ix–xii
http://dx.doi.org/10.1016/j.gtc.2012.08.011

appear to be critical in eliciting appropriate host responses, especially adaptive immunity. In fact, the gut microbial patterns associated with healthy vaginally born, breast-fed infants differ from those experiencing early life events such as birth by cesarean section, premature birth, lack of breast feeding, and treatment with antibiotics. These early life events, associated with altered microbial composition, are in turn associated with diseases of infancy, childhood, and later life, specifically immune-related conditions. Bifidobacteria and Lactobacilli are nonpathogenic bacteria that elicit beneficial host responses. The possible role of dysbiosis contributing to necrotizing enterocolitis, allergic diatheses, inflammatory diseases, metabolic syndrome, and obesity is discussed.

In a commentary on the safety of probiotics, Dr Shanahan offers information relating to the long record of safety, particularly related to lactobacilli and bifidobacteria. In fact, the risk appears to be low with currently available probiotic products. Safety should be considered on a strain-by-strain basis. Due caution should be accorded patients with indwelling central venous catheters, patients with synthetic cardiac valves, and those with profound immunosuppression.

Dr Isolauri has had a deep and abiding interest in the relationship of developing commensal bacteria and the association of allergic diatheses. She notes that gut microbiota composition can discriminate between allergic and healthy children, and this distinction may antedate clinical manifestations of disease. Bifidobacteria species are the major determinants of disease risk. Diminished presence of this species is associated with an elevated maternal BMI, weight gain during pregnancy, absence of breast feeding, and infant delivery by Caesarean section. Specific probiotics may modulate early microbial colonization, which represents the first intervention target in allergic disease, together with their ability to reverse the increased intestinal permeability characteristic of children with atopic eczema and food allergy. Probiotics also enhance gut-specific IgA responses, which are frequently defective in children with food allergy.

In their discussion of the treatment of necrotizing enterocolitis with probiotics, Drs Kriston Gangu Li and W. Allan Walker provide a concise update of this emerging field. This devastating intestinal disease of preterm infants is the most common gastrointestinal emergency in the neonatal intensive care unit and is associated with significant morbidity and mortality. Several functional characteristics of the immature intestine render the prematurely born infant ill-equipped to manage the multiple microbial challenges of extrauterine life. Probiotic bacteria have the ability to positively influence the process of bacterial colonization and modify immature intestinal immune responses, thereby decreasing the risk of developing necrotizing enterocolitis.Orally administered probiotics represent a promising new area of disease prevention.

Nucleic acid–based methods of analysis are widely used to determine and monitor the composition of microbes. This methodology facilitates logistical planning and execution of microbiota analysis for probiotic, clinical, and nutritional trials using human subjects. It is known that the impact of ingested probiotics is transient, being only detected in the feces while the probiotic is consumed. Drs Lawley and Tannock recommend that temporal studies of the microbiota be carried out, thus providing information regarding the stability/variability of microbiota compositions over time. The methods described in this article range from relatively simple (PCR) to the technically sophisticated (metatranscriptomics). Generally, a study could commence with a screening of samples to determine whether it will be worthwhile expending further time and money on an in-depth analysis. PCR-DGGE (TTGE) or FISH/FC are cost-effective choices for this purpose. An example of this comprehensive approach is provided by a study of the microbiota of ileoanal pouches.

Dr T.J. Borody is a leading investigator in the analysis and clinical application of fecal microbiota transplantation (FMT) in the treatment of gastrointestinal illnesses. This procedure has gained widespread recognition in light of the recent *Clostridium difficile* infection (CDI) epidemic in Canada, the United States, and Europe. The success rate, particularly in patients with recurrent CDI, has been dramatically impressive. This article provides an overview of the history of FMT, a review of FMT publications for CDI, and a discussion of the concept of the gut microbiota as a virtual organ. The authors then provide a rationale for FMT use in inflammatory bowel disease (IBD) and other possible emerging applications. Finally, a discussion is offered of how FMT is currently performed and how FMT may be performed in the future.

Dr Eamonn Quigley offers clinicians and investigators a concise, even-handed, in-depth analysis of the impact of probiotics on the various subdivisions of functional bowel disorders. An examination of the scientific basis for the use of probiotics in irritable bowel syndrome (IBS) reveals that new onset IBS may follow bacteriologically confirmed bacterial gastroenteritis. Postinfectious IBS may have long-lasting symptoms possibly based on low-grade inflammation and immune activation secondary to microbial–host engagement. Additionally, there is some evidence that inflammatory and immune processes may contribute to enteric neuromuscular dysfunction. Selected probiotics may be of value by exerting antibacterial (or antiviral) effects, increasing secretory IgA production, enhancing barrier function, preventing colonization by pathogenic bacteria, and reducing proinflammatory cytokine activity. There is some evidence that IBS patients may be deficient in strains and numbers of bifidobacteria and lactobacilli. Changes in the composition of microbiota with probiotics may produce beneficial metabolic functions by altering the efficiency of fermentation of complex carbohydrates, improving mucus barrier function, decreasing intraluminal gas production, and affecting motor dysfunction. Modulation of selected microbiota might benefit slow-transit constipated patients by accelerating motor transit. Specific bacteria, particularly selected bifidobacteria strains, have demonstrable impact on improving global symptoms of IBS. Probiotics in general seem to be most effective in reducing symptoms of bloating and flatulence. The role of probiotics in functional bowel disorders remains to be defined, requiring more long-term randomized, placebo-controlled studies defining optimal strain, dose, and formulation.

Dr G. Friedman offers corroborative evidence favoring the use of probiotics in the prevention of symptoms of antibiotic-associated diarrhea (AAD). Lactobacilli, *Saccharomyces boulardii*, and selected multistrain combinations, in appropriate dosages, are all clinically useful. The safety profile is generally acceptable particularly in view of the short-term use of an antibiotic when accompanied by a probiotic. *C difficile* colitis is the most common gastrointestinal infection, exceeding all other gastrointestinal infections combined. There has been a dramatic increase in CDI worldwide during the past decade. In-hospital morbidity and mortality, particularly among the elderly, are continuing to rise. In part, this has been related to a virulent strain, NAP1/B1/027, the virulence of which is enhanced by higher levels of toxins A and B, as well as by a greater tendency for recurrent CDI. Antibiotic therapy is a trigger precipitating AAD, which may lead to CDI. Selected probiotics have been effective in reducing AAD and preventing CDI.

Drs Fedorak and Demeria provide an in-depth analysis of probiotic bacteria in the prevention and treatment of IBD. There is little doubt that commensal bacteria play a significant role in the genesis of IBD in genetically predisposed patients. The precise mechanisms involved in the establishment and progression of IBD with respect to the host bacterial populations remain to be elucidated. There is good evidence supporting the use of probiotics in patients who have developed pouchitis. In patients with mild to moderate ulcerative colitis, probiotic preparations have similar efficacy to conventional treatment with aminosalicylates. Currently, there is insufficient evidence to support the use of probiotics in Crohn's disease. Well-designed, large, randomized controlled trials utilizing specific strains and appropriate dosages are required for probiotics to become mainstream therapy.

Gerald Friedman, MD, PhD, MS, FACP, MACG, AGAF
Department of Medicine
The Mount Sinai School of Medicine
New York, NY, USA

E-mail address:
gfmd379@gmail.com

Early Development of Intestinal Microbiota: Implications for Future Health

José M. Saavedra, MD[a,b,*], Anne M. Dattilo, PhD, RD[b]

KEYWORDS

- Microbiota • Intestine • Bacteria • Infant • Cesarean section • Prematurity

KEY POINTS

- Early acquisition and maintenance of a healthy intestinal microbiota is critical to the long-term health of the host; and the mechanisms through which this occurs are beginning to be elucidated.
- Factors that lead to alterations in microbial composition during infancy are associated with inadequate and inappropriate host immune responses, which lead to the development of disease.
- A greater understanding of these factors and of these mechanisms will unlock potential strategies to modulate the acquisition and maintenance of a human microbiota that maintains and promotes health.
- These strategies will be critical in battling the epidemic of noncommunicable immune-related diseases encountered in the modern world.

INTRODUCTION

The fetal gut lumen is devoid of any significant amounts of bacteria. But within a few hours after birth, the intestinal tract becomes colonized by microorganisms, collectively known as microbiota. This dramatic ecologic change in the gut lumen, from relative bacterial naiveté to exposure to billions of organisms of hundreds of species in a matter of days, is a key determinant in the development and maturation of gut barrier function mechanisms and the development and modulation of gut and systemic immune responses, primarily via its effect on gut-associated lymphoid tissue. The time of development, the microbial profile, and the diversity of this ecosystem seem to be critical in eliciting appropriate host responses, particularly adaptive immunity. A few specific bacterial genera and species seem to be important and relevant to

[a] Department of Pediatrics, Johns Hopkins University School of Medicine, 600 North Wolfe Street, Baltimore, MD 21287, USA; [b] Nestlé Nutrition, Medical Scientific and Regulatory Unit, 12 Vreeland Road, Florham Park, NJ 07932, USA
* Corresponding author. Nestle Nutrition, Medical Scientific and Regulatory Unit, 12 Vreeland Road, Florham Park, NJ 07932.
E-mail address: jose.saavedra@us.nestle.com

Gastroenterol Clin N Am 41 (2012) 717–731
http://dx.doi.org/10.1016/j.gtc.2012.08.001
0889-8553/12/$ – see front matter © 2012 Elsevier Inc. All rights reserved.

humans, eliciting beneficial immunologic host responses while not having significant pathogenic potential. Among these potentially "beneficial" bacteria are multiple nonpathogenic species of lactobacilli and bifidobacteria.

Inadequate or delayed bacterial acquisition and colonization can lead to aberrant microbial profiles, referred to by some as *dysbiosis*. This condition has been associated with a persistent Th2-dependent antibody profile, reduced inflammatory response, inadequate intestinal barrier function, deficient IgA synthesis, and poor oral tolerance,[1,2] and several pathologic conditions discussed later.

Microbiota composition in early infancy is characterized by microbial plasticity,[3] and several factors influence microbial composition in terms of rate of colonization, absolute bacterial counts, and microbial diversity. A vast literature base supports the influence that the mode of delivery (vaginal delivery vs cesarean section), dietary factors (breast-feeding vs infant formula), antibiotic exposure, and other environmental factors have on the development of microbiota. Emerging evidence also supports the influence of the prenatal environment and specific host–microbial interactions on microbiota composition in childhood,[4–6] and potentially beyond. This article describes the early gut microbiota, major determinants of acquisition and colonization, and selected health implications associated with changes or alterations in gut microbial populations.

COMPOSITION OF EARLY GUT MICROBIOTA

The bacterial content of infant feces can be identified within hours of birth and can contain greater than 10 (9) colony forming units (cfu) of bacteria per gram of stool within the first week.[7,8] During the first days of life, the bacterial colonization profile of a healthy, full-term infant is unstable and constitutes a limited array of organisms. Although bacteria vary along the intestinal tract and across the microstructures within the gut (eg, lumen, mucus layer, crypts, intestinal epithelial cells),[9] knowledge of the human infant gut microbiota is generally limited to assessments of microbial quality and quantity from stool samples. These samples reflect luminal colonic microbiota, and not necessarily the microbial composition of the proximal gut, particularly the small intestine, which includes a major component of gut-associated lymphoid tissue. Nevertheless, they are used as a practical surrogate for gastrointestinal microbiota.

Culture-based studies performed before 1990 provided initial estimates of number and types of gut microorganisms in infant stool. These assessments were the most practical techniques for understanding of the composition of microbiota at the time. These studies showed that the gastrointestinal tract of infants is first colonized by facultative anaerobes, such as *Escherichia coli* and Enterococci, at concentrations exceeding 10 (10) cfu/g feces.[7] Staphylococci and streptococci have also been isolated in significant concentrations.[10] Although the abundance of oxygen in the neonatal gut initially prevents the establishment of strict anaerobes, as the facultative anaerobic populations of bacteria expand and consume oxygen, an anaerobic environment is created that supports the growth of anaerobes. Thus, within the first week of life, *Bifidobacterium*, *Bacteroides*, and *Clostridium* spp have been isolated from at least half of healthy neonatal fecal samples at populations up to 10 (11) cfu/g,[7] and anaerobic species such as bifidobacteria have been recognized as the predominant component of the gastrointestinal bacterial mass.

The early selective culture-based assessments of microbiota led the way to more advanced qualification (better assessing microbial diversity or richness) and quantification (cfu per gram of stool) methods. To date only few studies have investigated infant microbiota after birth using these non–culture-based techniques.[11] The limited studies based on newer methodology have confirmed the dominance of bifidobacteria, clostridia, and bacteroides in early microbiota.[10,12–14]

Undoubtedly, some infant fecal bacteria have not yet been adequately cultured or speciated, but most of the gut microbiome is restricted to a small subset of phyla, genera, and culturable species of bacteria.[15] The gastrointestinal tract of humans is dominated almost entirely by only 4 of the recognized phyla of the bacterial kingdom: Firmicutes, Bacteroidetes, Actinobacteria, and Proteobacteria. Approximately 10% of infant samples in the first 2 months of life have been found to contain unidentified species through culture methods,[16] and some facultative bacteria[17] and anaerobes that are difficult to culture (eg, some *Ruminococcus* spp) have required DNA-based methods for identification.[16] However, most anaerobes in infants can be isolated through culture-based methods, with a sensitivity similar to that achieved with fluorescent in situ hybridization (FISH) or real-time polymerase chain reaction (PCR) (ie, fecal population $\geq$10 (3) cfu/g).[7] Thus, for infant microbiota assessments, culture-based studies still provide meaningful assessments of early infant microbiota.

DETERMINANTS OF INFANT MICROBIOTA

The establishment and composition of microbiota in the infant are influenced by numerous factors, including the prenatal-uterine environment, mode of birth, type of feeding, antibiotic use, and the immediate environment. Penders and colleagues[13] showed that full-term infants born vaginally at home who were exclusively breast-fed exhibited what some might consider the most beneficial gut microbiota, characterized by high numbers of *Bifidobacterium* spp and reduced abundance of *E coli* and *Clostridium difficile*. The major determinants of early acquisition of infant microbiota are reviewed in the following sections.

Prenatal Microbial Exposure

Based on the Barker hypothesis for the "developmental origins of adult disease,"[18] the prenatal environment has been implicated in the development of later disease, with examples such as low birth weight or prenatal undernutrition being linked to adult weight, type 2 diabetes, hypertension, and coronary artery disease. Maternal microbial exposure during gestation may have some direct effects on the fetus, and the infant's immune development[19] and long-term health.[20,21]

Direct bacterial exposure of the fetus through amniotic fluid, which is typically sterile, may have deleterious effects. Bacterial ribosomal DNA and bacteria from *Leptotrichia* spp and other related species have been identified in amniotic fluid of women in preterm labor,[20,21] and studies suggest that infant prematurity is positively associated with bacterial load, even in the absence of ruptured membranes.[20] Although the clinical significance of microbial identification in amniotic fluid has not been fully identified, investigators have suggested that microbes within amniotic fluid swallowed by the fetus could translocate through the intestinal epithelium and elicit inflammation, and potentially stimulate uterine contraction and premature delivery.[22]

On the other hand, maternal exposure to microbes during pregnancy seems to play a role in postnatal immune functioning, particularly regarding allergic disease.[23–25] Maternal prenatal exposure to household pets (cats and dogs) has been associated with lower cord blood IgE concentrations[26] and increased number and function of cord blood T-regulatory cells, and a lower incidence of allergic disease in children.[25,26] Mothers exposed to farms and farm animals during pregnancy were also less likely to have children who developed allergies and asthma.[23,27] The degree and diversity of maternal exposure to microbes may also have an impact. Higher levels of innate immune components, Toll-like receptors (TLR2, TLR4, and CD14), have been identified in children whose mothers were exposed to stables during the prenatal period, and for every extra farm-associated animal species a mother encountered, expression levels increased by up to 1.16-fold.[23]

Evidence shows the potential of small, yet immunogenic, allergen fragments to cross the placenta and prime naïve fetal T cells, resulting in a form of natural immunity during gestation. These allergens, in concert with maternal immunologic responses to microbial exposure, seem to shape the fetal immunologic environment in a way that can affect postnatal predisposition to disease.[28]

Mode of Birth

During vaginal birth, microbes from the birth canal, the perineum, and the mother's skin constitute the first bacterial inocula for gastrointestinal luminal colonization. Thus, the infant's early microbiota profile is similar to the mother's vaginal and fecal microbes.[5,29] Although individual variation exists, facultative anaerobic E coli and Streptococcus spp tend to dominate in infant stool in the first 2 to 3 days after birth. However, within a few days, anaerobic genera, such as bifidobacteria and bacteroides (which have been associated with beneficial effects, including down-regulation of inflammatory responses),[30,31] become quantitatively more important in the infant stool of vaginally born infants.

In contrast, infants born by cesarean section (CS) show delayed colonization and lack of microbial diversity.[5,32] Differences in composition of microbiota during the first days, months, and years of life have been reported for infants delivered by CS compared with infants born vaginally.[13,29,33–36] Often, the early microbiota of infants delivered by CS consists of species found within the bacterial hospital environment, including reduced levels of strict anaerobes such as bifidobacteria.[37,38] Compared with vaginally born infants, those born by CS tend to harbor higher stool quantities and/or increased prevalence of Staphylococcus spp, Streptococcus spp,[28] C difficile, klebsiella, and enterobacteria, and a reduced prevalence of bacteroides,[24,32,37] and reduced or delayed colonization with bifidobacteria and lactobacilli.[33,34,39] These altered patterns have been documented up to 7 years of age.[36]

Adequate data are not available to compare microbiota of infants delivered by CS at the time of membrane rupture and those with early membrane rupture who were allowed some exposure to vaginal flora. Investigators have suggested that physical passage of the infant through the birth canal may be more important than the presence or duration of rupture of membranes in determining early microbial composition.[11]

In summary, infants born by CS experience significant deviation from the normal pattern of microbiota acquisition, and develop gastrointestinal microbial profiles distinctly different from those of infants born vaginally. This "aberrant" type of intestinal microbiota has been implicated in altered immunologic host responses that could lead to immune-related conditions in later life. CS delivery has been identified as an independent risk factor for the development of several conditions, including allergic disease, including asthma, and gastroenteritis in later childhood.[40–42] Meta-analysis findings from 23 studies on the association between mode of birth and allergic disease showed a 20% increase in the development of asthma in children delivered by CS compared with those delivered vaginally.[42] A more than 7-fold increase in risk of allergy has been reported for children born to mothers with a history of allergy who were also delivered by CS. These relationships remained significant after adjusting for confounding variables, including short-term breast-feeding.[43]

Of even greater interest is the increasing identification of CS as an independent risk factor of immune-related conditions other than allergic disorders. Various studies have investigated a relationship between CS delivery and type 1 diabetes. A recent meta-analysis of these studies showed a 20% increase in the risk of childhood-onset type 1 diabetes associated with CS delivery that was not explained by known confounders.[44] In a large retrospective, multicenter, case-control study, a significantly enhanced likelihood of being born by CS was found in children with celiac disease compared with control subjects.[45] In this cohort CS delivery was not found to be associated with Crohn disease or ulcerative colitis.

Finally, recent studies suggest that obesity and metabolic syndrome may be associated with changes in microbiota.[46,47] A prospective cohort study showed that infants delivered by CS had 2-fold higher odds of obesity at age 3 years, even after adjusting for maternal body mass index, birthweight, and other confounding variables.[48] Although causality and potential mechanisms remain to be elucidated, increasing evidence shows a relationship between the establishment of microbiota in early life and subsequent phenotypic manifestations in the host, including changes in adiposity and related metabolic alterations.

The increasing recognition of CS as a risk factor for chronic conditions that manifest themselves far beyond the perinatal period should foster increased awareness of these risks, and serve as additional argument against non–medically indicated CS.

Dietary Intake

Diet is one of the most important determinants of microbial diversity in the gut.[13] In the full-term breast-fed infant, anaerobic bacteria from the genus *Bifidobacterium* begin to colonize the gut within the first week of life. Bifidobacteria can constitute more than 60% of the fecal bacteria in breast-fed infants within 6 days of nursing,[49] and up to 72% by the third week of exclusive breast-feeding.[9] Factors likely responsible for a strong dominance of bifidobacteria in the stool of breast-fed infants include the presence of multiple *Bifidobacterium* spp in maternal milk that provide a constant inocula to the infant,[50–53] and several breast milk components, including galacto-oligosaccharides, which selectively foster the growth of bifidobacteria in the gut.

Compared with breast-fed infants, formula-fed babies are less frequently colonized with bifidobacteria, tend to have bifidobacteria in lower numbers, and are more often colonized with potentially pathogenic species of enterococci, coliforms, and clostridia. Specifically, populations of *E coli*, *C difficile*, and bacteroides have been rather consistently reported as being more prevalent or reaching higher counts in stool from formula-fed infants.[13,49,54]

Although limited studies have reported no significant difference in the numbers of bifidobacteria in stools of exclusively formula- or breast-fed infants,[54] Klaassens and colleagues[55] identified that the functional gene expression and type of bifidobacteria present in infant stool was shown to differ with mode of feeding. Moreover, the widespread inclusion of lactose and compounds similar to bifidogenic human milk oligosaccharides, such as galacto-oligosaccharides,[56] in commercial formulas may account for some less-than-expected differences in stool microbiota of formula-fed infants.

By approximately 2 years of age, when children are consuming an adult-type diet, the gut community begins to resemble that of an adult-like microbiota. Once established, both the microbiota[4–6] and caloric contribution of various food groups[57] in late infancy remain reasonably stable. However, clinically induced variations in dietary macronutrient contribution have been associated with changes in microbiota. Increased numbers of Firmicutes and reduced numbers of Bacteroidetes[58–60] and bifidobacteria[59] have been documented with high-fat feeding in both animal and human studies, although long-term follow-up studies are not available to determine if these changes persist.

Antibiotic Exposure

Antibiotic use can significantly alter the composition of intestinal microbiota,[61] and may do so in specific ways in infants. Dramatic decreases in microbial diversity with antibiotic administration during the first year of life have been reported[5] in term infants. Administration of antibiotics (primarily cephalosporins or oral amoxicillin) in the first months of life resulted in reduced numbers of fecal bifidobacteria and bacteroides and overgrowth of *C difficile*.[13] In premature infants, the duration of antibiotic treatment in the first month of life has been shown to correlate with decreased bacterial diversity.[62] Enterococci populations were increased 1 month after a 4-day treatment of broad-spectrum antibiotics in neonates.[63]

Unlike adults, who may return quickly to pretreatment microbiota after cessation of antibiotic treatment, the effect of antibiotics on infant's microbiota may affect immune homeostasis and create immediate susceptibility to disease[61] with long-lasting consequences. Antibiotic exposure during the first year of life has been identified as an independent risk factor for wheezing,[64–66] and meta-analyses identify it as a risk factor for childhood asthma.[65] Early antibiotic exposure has been associated with increased risk of childhood atopy,[67] and increased frequency of antibiotic use also correlated with atopic risk.[68] These findings underscore the importance of the initial period of host bacterial experience, and a critical window in which aberrations in colonization patterns may induce long-term changes in microbiota and in immunologic responses, with long-term consequences.

Other Factors

The immediate environment in early life can also affect microbiota composition. The gut is colonized with a only a small number of bacterial species in hospitalized, premature infants; lactobacilli and bifidobacteria are rarely identified in microbiota.[32] Hospitalization of neonates after birth for as little as 4 days has been associated with decreased prevalence of bifidobacteria and higher *C difficile* colonization rates.[13]

Finally, the role of the individual, the unique host harboring this complex ecosystem of bacteria, cannot be underestimated. Individual differences in the luminal environment provided to the microbiota can also affect its composition. Differences in factors such as oxygen tension and lumen redox potential, pH, the composition of digestive enzymes, biliary secretions, mucus and mucin, and IgA production are all specific and phenotypically unique to each individual host, and these variations can modulate the microbiota in ways that are only beginning to be understood.[69]

MICROBIOTA COMPOSITION AND ASSOCIATIONS WITH DISEASE

There is increasing recognition that disturbed acquisition and composition of microbiota during early infancy may be linked to the risk of developing disease later in life.

Atopic Diseases

Much of the evidence for the link between early microbial populations and subsequent development of immune disorders come from studies of atopic disease, and the evidence is strong for a link between early gastrointestinal colonization and subsequent development of allergic manifestations, such as eczema[16,38,70–73] and asthma.[38,74,75] Evaluation of approximately 1000 stool samples of 1-month-old infants identified a high prevalence of *E coli* associated with later development of eczema, and those with a high count of *C difficile* were associated with a higher risk of eczema, recurrent wheeze, allergic sensitization, and atopic dermatitis.[38] In addition, allergic infants and children were found to have less colonization with lactobacilli and bifidobacteria, and the prevalence of colonization with bifidobacteria in infants who developed allergy during the first 2 years of life was less than for those that did not develop atopy.[76] In addition to decreased bifidobacteria, allergic infants were colonized less often with *Bacteroides* spp and more often with *Staphylococcus aureus*.[75,77] Furthermore, a reduced ratio of bifidobacteria to clostridium in early gut microbiota has been reported to precede allergic disease.[75]

Overall, a more diverse early gut microbiota is more common among nonallergic infants than in those with allergy,[16] yet whether low diversity of the gut microbiota in infancy is more important than the prevalence of specific bacterial taxa in the development of allergic disease has been a matter of debate. Infants with sensitization or eczema were reported to have fewer microbial peaks/bands than healthy infants,[16,70,78] without regard to specific microbes. High-throughput 16S-based molecular microbiology recently confirmed these previous findings.[79] More recent results indicate that low intestinal microbial diversity during first month of life was associated with subsequent atopic eczema and may be more relevant than any specific bacteria.[79] One proposed rationale for the importance of microbial diversity is based on the assumption that the gut immune system reacts to exposure to new bacterial antigens, and these repeated exposures of various microbes would enhance the development of immune regulation.[80]

In summary, differences in microbiota among infants developing allergy and those who do not suggest that factors in early life that alter gut microbial composition may be a determinant in the later development of this immunologic disease. In fact, cesarean birth, antibiotic use, and formula-feeding (rather than breast-feeding), all of which are associated with the altered patterns of microbiota, are also independent risk factors for allergic conditions.

Obesity and Metabolic Syndrome

Low-grade systemic inflammation has been associated with overweight, obesity, and disorders directly linked to adiposity, such as insulin resistance and type 2 diabetes. Microbiota has been suggested to be a contributing factor in the development of some of these metabolic disorders.[81] Several studies have shown that, compared with lean individuals, those who are obese harbor a greater concentration of Firmicutes[82,83] and have an exaggerated shift in the ratio of Firmicutes to Bacteroidetes (from 3:1 to 35:1), 2 of the major phyla present in the adult human gastrointestinal tract.[84] This altered bacterial quantity has been implicated in obesity development through its effects on increasing energy harvest from food and its interactions with epithelial and endocrine cells that promote insulin resistance and inflammation and increase adipocyte generation.[85–87] Thus, microbiota, influenced by acquisition and composition in early life, may play a significant role in the development of overweight or obesity.

One recent prospective trial of 138 infants identified (by culture on selective media) that a microbiota with high *Bacteroides fragilis* and low staphylococcus concentrations in infants between the age of 3 weeks and 1 year was associated with a higher risk of obesity during preschool age.[88] A separate longitudinal study of microbiota composition during infancy (at 6 and 12 months) and 7 years later examined 25 children who became overweight/obese by age 7 and 24 children who remained normal weight. Results from FISH analysis and quantitative PCR showed that the amount of fecal bifidobacteria was greater and the concentration of *S aureus* lower in children remaining normal weight compared with those who later became overweight.[89] The authors proposed that protection from obesity noted with higher bifidobacteria may be partly mediated by its potential anti-inflammatory effects, whereas *S aureus* may act as a trigger of low-grade inflammation, contributing to difficulty with weight management. A third study that examined microbiota composition during infancy (3 weeks and 3 months of age) through FISH analyses identified a trend toward reduced bifidobacteria counts in 3-month fecal samples and overweight status in children at age 10 years, compared with their normal-weight counterparts.[90]

Mechanistic studies and a more comprehensive understanding of obesity and metabolic disorders in relation to gut microbiota are necessary. Nevertheless, the fact that by 2 years of age the microbiota reaches a stable compositional state,[4–6] and that adiposity measures starting at 2 years of age track into later childhood,[91] provides additional impetus for research in this area.

Necrotizing Enterocolitis

Premature infants are a population at particular risk of developing an aberrant microbiota composition. They are often born by CS, most are administered antibiotics, they are infrequently breast-fed, and their first microbial surrounding is the hospital environment. As would be expected, premature infants have delayed patterns of colonization, decreased microbial diversity, increased numbers of potentially pathogenic bacteria, and decreased colonization with bifidobacteria. These deviations are often identified in premature infants who develop necrotizing enterocolitis (NEC). Specific strains of klebsiella, enterobacteria, or *E coli* in microbiota have been shown to precede the development of NEC, and fecal colonization with enterococcus and *Candida albicans* has been identified more frequently in symptomatic infants than controls.[92]

Infantile Colic

Potential mechanisms implicated in the occurrence of bouts of excessive and inconsolable crying in infants include behavioral, digestive, and gastrointestinal motility factors. Recently, differences in gut microbiota have been reported between infants with symptoms of colic and those without.[93–95] Infants with colic seem to harbor more gas-producing bacteria (eg, *E coli*) and be less frequently colonized by non–gas producing microbes (eg, lactobacilli and bifidobacteria).[93] Other recent studies identified that colicky infants were more likely to have a restricted bacterial diversity and were more frequently colonized with coliforms such as *Klebsiella* spp, *Enterococcus* spp, *and E coli* than age-matched controls[96]; these findings remained when differences in exposure to antibiotics and types of feeding were considered. Whether abnormal microbiota is the cause of infantile colic or the result of intestinal luminal factors such as inflammation has yet to be determined. Similarly, whether an association exists between intestinal bacteria and other functional disorders, such as functional abdominal pain and irritable bowel syndrome, awaits additional investigation.

Crohn Disease

A decreased quantity and biodiversity of bacteria within the Firmicutes phylum has been repeatedly observed in patients with Crohn disease (CD),[97,98] and further evidence of this comes from a recent study with twins designed to consider genetic influences.[99] When comparing discordant and concordant twin pairs, regardless of disease state, the intestinal microbial composition showed a dramatically lower abundance of *Faecalibacterium prausnitzii* and increased abundance of *E coli* in twins with CD, compared with healthy co-twins and those with CD localized in the colon. The reduction in *F prausnitzii*, a major member of the Firmicutes phylum, which has anti-inflammatory properties, was associated with an increased risk of recurrence of ileal CD. Using a variety of assessment methodologies, decreased bifidobacteria and lactobacilli have been found in adults[100] and children[101] with CD.

In summary, several pathologic conditions are related to alterations in microbiota composition when compared with healthy individuals. Although most of these observations of various dysbiosis linked to disease do not prove causality, they indicate a close relationship between intestinal microbiota and numerous gut-barrier, immune, and possibly also metabolic functions of the host, which argues strongly for a major role of gastrointestinal microbes in the development and modulation of these disorders. Additional evidence of this is derived from transplantation experiments in which the altered microbiota from a diseased animal was provided to a germ-free healthy recipient; several disease phenotypes could be transferred by the microbiota. These include excess adiposity, metabolic syndrome, and colitis.[60,102,103] In humans, fecal transplantation with donor fecal flora, have shown some success in treatment of Crohn's disease, *C difficile*–associated diarrhea, ulcerative colitis, and chronic constipation.[104–106]

Finally, the possibility of beneficially affecting the host's health through modulating the composition of the intestinal bacterial composition via ingestion of bacteria, the concept of probiotics, has resulted in an explosion of research over the past 2 decades. The use of specific bacteria, particularly species from the genus *Bifidobacterium* and *Lactobacillus*, has been shown with varying but increasing levels of documentation to have both preventive and therapeutic benefits in several conditions, including allergic conditions, inflammatory gastrointestinal disorders, NEC, and functional gastrointestinal disorders, including infantile colic,[107,108] all of which are associated to alterations in the microbiota. Although this topic is beyond the scope of this review, the effects of orally administered bacteria, which change the gastrointestinal ecosystem and improve those same conditions associated to altered patterns of gastrointestinal microbiota, provide additional evidence of a direct causal link between the microbiota and host health.

SUMMARY

It is unquestionable today that early acquisition and maintenance of a healthy intestinal microbiota is critical to the long-term health of the host, and the mechanisms through which this occurs are beginning to be elucidated. Factors that lead to alterations in microbial composition during infancy are associated with inadequate and inappropriate host immune responses, which lead to the development of disease. A greater understanding of these factors and mechanisms will unlock potential strategies to modulate the acquisition and maintenance of a human microbiota that maintains and promotes health. These strategies will be critical in battling the epidemic of noncommunicable immune-related diseases encountered in the modern world.

REFERENCES

1. Sjogren YM, Tomicic S, Lundberg A, et al. Influence of early gut microbiota on the maturation of childhood mucosal and systemic immune responses. Clin Exp Allergy 2009;39:1842–51.
2. Sudo N, Sawamura S, Tanaka K, et al. The requirement of intestinal bacterial flora for the development of an IgE production system fully susceptible to oral tolerance induction. J Immunol 1997;159:1739–45.
3. Krajmalnik-Brown R, Ilhan ZE, Kang DW, et al. Effects of gut microbes on nutrient absorption and energy regulation. Nutr Clin Pract 2012;27:201–14.

4. O'Toole PW, Claesson MJ. Gut microbiota: changes throughout the lifespan from infancy to elderly. Int Dairy J 2010;20:281–91.
5. Palmer C, Bik EM, DiGiulio DB, et al. Development of the human infant intestinal microbiota. PLoS Biol 2007;5:e177.
6. Ringel-Kulka T. Targeting the intestinal microbiota in the pediatric population: a clinical perspective. Nutr Clin Pract 2012;27:226–34.
7. Adlerberth I, Wold AE. Establishment of the gut microbiota in Western infants. Acta Paediatr 2009;98:229–38.
8. Bezirtzoglou E, Tsiotsias A, Welling GW. Microbiota profile in feces of breast- and formula-fed newborns by using fluorescence in situ hybridization (FISH). Anaerobe 2011;17:478–82.
9. Lievin-Le Moal V, Servin AL. The front line of enteric host defense against unwel-come intrusion of harmful microorganisms: mucins, antimicrobial peptides, and microbiota. Clin Microbiol Rev 2006;19:315–37.
10. Bezirtzoglou E, Stavropoulou E. Immunology and probiotic impact of the newborn and young children intestinal microflora. Anaerobe 2011;17:369–74.
11. Neu J, Rushing J. Cesarean versus vaginal delivery: long-term infant outcomes and the hygiene hypothesis. Clin Perinatol 2011;38:321–31.
12. Hopkins MJ, Macfarlane GT, Furrie E, et al. Characterisation of intestinal bacteria in infant stools using real-time PCR and northern hybridisation anal-yses. FEMS Microbiol Ecol 2005;54:77–85.
13. Penders J, Thijs C, Vink C, et al. Factors influencing the composition of the intes-tinal microbiota in early infancy. Pediatrics 2006;118:511–21.
14. Wang M, Ahrne S, Antonsson M, et al. T-RFLP combined with principal compo-nent analysis and 16S rRNA gene sequencing: an effective strategy for compar-ison of fecal microbiota in infants of different ages. J Microbiol Methods 2004;59: 53–69.
15. Hattori M, Taylor TD. The human intestinal microbiome: a new frontier of human biology. DNA Res 2009;16:1–12.
16. Wang M, Karlsson C, Olsson C, et al. Reduced diversity in the early fecal microbiota of infants with atopic eczema. J Allergy Clin Immunol 2008;121: 129–34.
17. Hayashi H, Takahashi R, Nishi T, et al. Molecular analysis of jejunal, ileal, caecal and recto-sigmoidal human colonic microbiota using 16S rRNA gene libraries and terminal restriction fragment length polymorphism. J Med Microbiol 2005; 54:1093–101.
18. Barker DJ. The fetal and infant origins of adult disease. BMJ 1990;301:1111.
19. Kaplan JL, Shi HN, Walker WA. The role of microbes in developmental immuno-logic programming. Pediatr Res 2011;69:465–72.
20. DiGiulio DB, Romero R, Amogan HP, et al. Microbial prevalence, diversity and abundance in amniotic fluid during preterm labor: a molecular and culture-based investigation. PLoS One 2008;3:e3056.
21. Han YW, Shen T, Chung P, et al. Uncultivated bacteria as etiologic agents of intra-amniotic inflammation leading to preterm birth. J Clin Microbiol 2009;47: 38–47.
22. Neu J, Young CM, Mai V. The developing intestinal microbiome: implications for the neonate. In: Cleason CA, Devaskar S, editors. Avery's diseases of the newborn. 9th edition. Philadelphia: Elsevier; 2012. p. 1016–21.
23. Ege MJ, Bieli C, Frei R, et al. Prenatal farm exposure is related to the expression of receptors of the innate immunity and to atopic sensitization in school-age chil-dren. J Allergy Clin Immunol 2006;117:817–23.

24. Penders J, Stobberingh EE, Thijs C, et al. Molecular fingerprinting of the intestinal microbiota of infants in whom atopic eczema was or was not developing. Clin Exp Allergy 2006;36:1602–8.

25. Wegienka G, Havstad S, Zoratti EM, et al. Regulatory T cells in prenatal blood samples: variability with pet exposure and sensitization. J Reprod Immunol 2009;81:74–81.

26. Aichbhaumik N, Zoratti EM, Strickler R, et al. Prenatal exposure to household pets influences fetal immunoglobulin E production. Clin Exp Allergy 2008;38: 1787–94.

27. Schaub B, Liu J, Hoppler S, et al. Maternal farm exposure modulates neonatal immune mechanisms through regulatory T cells. J Allergy Clin Immunol 2009; 123:774–82.

28. Fujimura KE, Slusher NA, Cabana MD, et al. Role of the gut microbiota in defining human health. Expert Rev Anti Infect Ther 2010;8:435–54.

29. Dominguez-Bello MG, Costello EK, Contreras M, et al. Delivery mode shapes the acquisition and structure of the initial microbiota across multiple body habitats in newborns. Proc Natl Acad Sci U S A 2010;107:11971–5.

30. Corr SC, Hill C, Gahan CG. Understanding the mechanisms by which probiotics inhibit gastrointestinal pathogens. Adv Food Nutr Res 2009;56:1–15.

31. Kelly D, Campbell JI, King TP, et al. Commensal anaerobic gut bacteria attenuate inflammation by regulating nuclear-cytoplasmic shuttling of PPAR-gamma and RelA. Nat Immunol 2004;5:104–12.

32. Fanaro S, Chierici R, Guerrini P, et al. Intestinal microflora in early infancy: composition and development. Acta Paediatr Suppl 2003;91:48–55.

33. Biasucci G, Benenati B, Morelli L, et al. Cesarean delivery may affect the early biodiversity of intestinal bacteria. J Nutr 2008;138:1796S–800S.

34. Biasucci G, Rubini M, Riboni S, et al. Mode of delivery affects the bacterial community in the newborn gut. Early Hum Dev 2010;86(Suppl 1):13–5.

35. Gronlund MM, Lehtonen OP, Eerola E, et al. Fecal microflora in healthy infants born by different methods of delivery: permanent changes in intestinal flora after cesarean delivery. J Pediatr Gastroenterol Nutr 1999;28:19–25.

36. Salminen S, Gibson GR, McCartney AL, et al. Influence of mode of delivery on gut microbiota composition in seven year old children. Gut 2004;53: 1388–9.

37. Adlerberth I, Strachan DP, Matricardi PM, et al. Gut microbiota and development of atopic eczema in 3 European birth cohorts. J Allergy Clin Immunol 2007;120: 343–50.

38. Penders J, Thijs C, van den Brandt PA, et al. Gut microbiota composition and development of atopic manifestations in infancy: the KOALA Birth Cohort Study. Gut 2007;56:661–7.

39. Huurre A, Kalliomaki M, Rautava S, et al. Mode of delivery - effects on gut microbiota and humoral immunity. Neonatology 2008;93:236–40.

40. Bager P, Melbye M, Rostgaard K, et al. Mode of delivery and risk of allergic rhinitis and asthma. J Allergy Clin Immunol 2003;111:51–6.

41. Bager P, Wohlfahrt J, Westergaard T. Caesarean delivery and risk of atopy and allergic disease: meta-analyses. Clin Exp Allergy 2008;38:634–42.

42. Thavagnanam S, Fleming J, Bromley A, et al. A meta-analysis of the association between Caesarean section and childhood asthma. Clin Exp Allergy 2008;38: 629–33.

43. Eggesbo M, Botten G, Stigum H, et al. Is delivery by cesarean section a risk factor for food allergy? J Allergy Clin Immunol 2003;112:420–6.

44. Cardwell CR, Stene LC, Joner G, et al. Caesarean section is associated with an increased risk of childhood-onset type 1 diabetes mellitus: a meta-analysis of observational studies. Diabetologia 2008;51:726–35.
45. Decker E, Engelmann G, Findeisen A, et al. Cesarean delivery is associated with celiac disease but not inflammatory bowel disease in children. Pediatrics 2010; 125:e1433–40.
46. Tilg H, Kaser A. Gut microbiome, obesity, and metabolic dysfunction. J Clin Invest 2011;121:2126–32.
47. Zhou L, He G, Zhang J, et al. Risk factors of obesity in preschool children in an urban area in China. Eur J Pediatr 2011;170:1401–6.
48. Huh SY, Rifas-Shiman SL, Zera CA, et al. Delivery by caesarean section and risk of obesity in preschool age children: a prospective cohort study. Arch Dis Child 2012;97(7):610–6.
49. Harmsen HJ, Wildeboer-Veloo AC, Raangs GC, et al. Analysis of intestinal flora development in breast-fed and formula-fed infants by using molecular identification and detection methods. J Pediatr Gastroenterol Nutr 2000;30: 61–7.
50. Gronlund MM, Gueimonde M, Laitinen K, et al. Maternal breast-milk and intestinal bifidobacteria guide the compositional development of the Bifidobacterium microbiota in infants at risk of allergic disease. Clin Exp Allergy 2007;37: 1764–72.
51. Gueimonde M, Laitinen K, Salminen S, et al. Breast milk: a source of bifidobacteria for infant gut development and maturation? Neonatology 2007;92:64–6.
52. Martin R, Jimenez E, Heilig H, et al. Isolation of bifidobacteria from breast milk and assessment of the bifidobacterial population by PCR-denaturing gradient gel electrophoresis and quantitative real-time PCR. Appl Environ Microbiol 2009;75:965–9.
53. Perez PF, Dore J, Leclerc M, et al. Bacterial imprinting of the neonatal immune system: lessons from maternal cells? Pediatrics 2007;119:e724–32.
54. Penders J, Vink C, Driessen C, et al. Quantification of Bifidobacterium spp., Escherichia coli and Clostridium difficile in faecal samples of breast-fed and formula-fed infants by real-time PCR. FEMS Microbiol Lett 2005;243:141–7.
55. Klaassens ES, Boesten RJ, Haarman M, et al. Mixed-species genomic microarray analysis of fecal samples reveals differential transcriptional responses of bifidobacteria in breast- and formula-fed infants. Appl Environ Microbiol 2009; 75:2668–76.
56. Fanaro S, Marten B, Bagna R, et al. Galacto-oligosaccharides are bifidogenic and safe at weaning: a double-blind randomized multicenter study. J Pediatr Gastroenterol Nutr 2009;48:82–8.
57. Deming DM, Reidy KC, Briefel RR, et al. The Feeding Infants and Toddlers Study (FITS) 2008: dramatic changes in the amount and quality of vegetables in the diet occur after the first year of life (abstract). Faseb J 2012;26:374.4.
58. Hildebrandt MA, Hoffmann C, Sherrill-Mix SA, et al. High-fat diet determines the composition of the murine gut microbiome independently of obesity. Gastroenterology 2009;137:1716–24.
59. Nadal I, Santacruz A, Marcos A, et al. Shifts in clostridia, bacteroides and immunoglobulin-coating fecal bacteria associated with weight loss in obese adolescents. Int J Obes (Lond) 2009;33:758–67.
60. Turnbaugh PJ, Backhed F, Fulton L, et al. Diet-induced obesity is linked to marked but reversible alterations in the mouse distal gut microbiome. Cell Host Microbe 2008;3:213–23.

61. Willing BP, Russell SL, Finlay BB. Shifting the balance: antibiotic effects on host-microbiota mutualism. Nat Rev Microbiol 2011;9:233–43.

62. Magne F, Suau A, Pochart P, et al. Fecal microbial community in preterm infants. J Pediatr Gastroenterol Nutr 2005;41:386–92.

63. Tanaka S, Kobayashi T, Songjinda P, et al. Influence of antibiotic exposure in the early postnatal period on the development of intestinal microbiota. FEMS Immunol Med Microbiol 2009;56:80–7.

64. Alm B, Erdes L, Mollborg P, et al. Neonatal antibiotic treatment is a risk factor for early wheezing. Pediatrics 2008;121:697–702.

65. Marra F, Lynd L, Coombes M, et al. Does antibiotic exposure during infancy lead to development of asthma?: a systematic review and metaanalysis. Chest 2006; 129:610–8.

66. Verhulst SL, Vael C, Beunckens C, et al. A longitudinal analysis on the association between antibiotic use, intestinal microflora, and wheezing during the first year of life. J Asthma 2008;45:828–32.

67. Johnson CC, Ownby DR, Alford SH, et al. Antibiotic exposure in early infancy and risk for childhood atopy. J Allergy Clin Immunol 2005;115:1218–24.

68. Watanabe J, Fujiwara R, Sasajima N, et al. Administration of antibiotics during infancy promoted the development of atopic dermatitis-like skin lesions in NC/Nga mice. Biosci Biotechnol Biochem 2010;74:358–63.

69. Bevins CL, Salzman NH. The potter's wheel: the host's role in sculpting its microbiota. Cell Mol Life Sci 2011;68:3675–85.

70. Forno E, Onderdonk AB, McCracken J, et al. Diversity of the gut microbiota and eczema in early life. Clin Mol Allergy 2008;6:11.

71. Gore C, Munro K, Lay C, et al. *Bifidobacterium pseudocatenulatum* is associated with atopic eczema: a nested case-control study investigating the fecal microbiota of infants. J Allergy Clin Immunol 2008;121:135–40.

72. Hong PY, Lee BW, Aw M, et al. Comparative analysis of fecal microbiota in infants with and without eczema. PLoS One 2010;5:e9964.

73. Kirjavainen PV, Arvola T, Salminen SJ, et al. Aberrant composition of gut microbiota of allergic infants: a target of bifidobacterial therapy at weaning? Gut 2002; 51:51–5.

74. Devereux G. The increase in the prevalence of asthma and allergy: food for thought. Nat Rev Immunol 2006;6:869–74.

75. Kalliomaki M, Kirjavainen P, Eerola E, et al. Distinct patterns of neonatal gut microflora in infants in whom atopy was and was not developing. J Allergy Clin Immunol 2001;107:129–34.

76. Bjorksten B, Sepp E, Julge K, et al. Allergy development and the intestinal microflora during the first year of life. J Allergy Clin Immunol 2001;108:516–20.

77. Bjorksten B, Naaber P, Sepp E, et al. The intestinal microflora in allergic Estonian and Swedish 2-year-old children. Clin Exp Allergy 1999;29:342–6.

78. Bisgaard H, Li N, Bonnelykke K, et al. Reduced diversity of the intestinal microbiota during infancy is associated with increased risk of allergic disease at school age. J Allergy Clin Immunol 2011;128:646–52.

79. Abrahamsson TR, Jakobsson HE, Andersson AF, et al. Low diversity of the gut microbiota in infants with atopic eczema. J Allergy Clin Immunol 2012;129: 434–40, 440.e1–2.

80. Holt PG. Postnatal maturation of immune competence during infancy and childhood. Pediatr Allergy Immunol 1995;6:59–70.

81. Cani PD, Delzenne NM. The role of the gut microbiota in energy metabolism and metabolic disease. Curr Pharm Des 2009;15:1546–58.

82. De Filippo C, Cavalieri D, Di PM, et al. Impact of diet in shaping gut microbiota revealed by a comparative study in children from Europe and rural Africa. Proc Natl Acad Sci U S A 2010;107:14691–6.

83. Ley RE, Backhed F, Turnbaugh P, et al. Obesity alters gut microbial ecology. Proc Natl Acad Sci U S A 2005;102:11070–5.

84. Ley RE, Turnbaugh PJ, Klein S, et al. Microbial ecology: human gut microbes associated with obesity. Nature 2006;444:1022–3.

85. Ley RE. Obesity and the human microbiome. Curr Opin Gastroenterol 2010;26: 5–11.

86. Reinhardt C, Reigstad CS, Backhed F. Intestinal microbiota during infancy and its implications for obesity. J Pediatr Gastroenterol Nutr 2009;48:249–56.

87. Turnbaugh PJ, Ley RE, Mahowald MA, et al. An obesity-associated gut microbiome with increased capacity for energy harvest. Nature 2006;444:1027–31.

88. Vael C, Verhulst SL, Nelen V, et al. Intestinal microflora and body mass index during the first three years of life: an observational study. Gut Pathog 2011;3:8.

89. Kalliomaki M, Collado MC, Salminen S, et al. Early differences in fecal microbiota composition in children may predict overweight. Am J Clin Nutr 2008;87:534–8.

90. Luoto R, Kalliomaki M, Laitinen K, et al. Initial dietary and microbiological environments deviate in normal-weight compared to overweight children at 10 years of age. J Pediatr Gastroenterol Nutr 2011;52:90–5.

91. Dattilo AM, Birch L, Krebs NF, et al. Need for early interventions in the prevention of pediatric overweight: a review and upcoming directions. J Obes 2012;2012: 1–18.

92. Hallstrom M, Eerola E, Vuento R, et al. Effects of mode of delivery and necrotising enterocolitis on the intestinal microflora in preterm infants. Eur J Clin Microbiol Infect Dis 2004;23:463–70.

93. Savino F, Cresi F, Pautasso S, et al. Intestinal microflora in breastfed colicky and non-colicky infants. Acta Paediatr 2004;93:825–9.

94. Savino F, Cordisco L, Tarasco V, et al. Molecular identification of coliform bacteria from colicky breastfed infants. Acta Paediatr 2009;98:1582–8.

95. Savino F, Cordisco L, Tarasco V, et al. Lactobacillus reuteri DSM 17938 in infantile colic: a randomized, double-blind, placebo-controlled trial. Pediatrics 2010; 126:e526–33.

96. Savino F, Cordisco L, Tarasco V, et al. Antagonistic effect of Lactobacillus strains against gas-producing coliforms isolated from colicky infants. BMC Microbiol 2011;11:157.

97. De Cruz P, Prideaux L, Wagner J, et al. Characterization of the gastrointestinal microbiota in health and inflammatory bowel disease. Inflamm Bowel Dis 2012;18:372–90.

98. Sokol H, Pigneur B, Watterlot L, et al. Faecalibacterium prausnitzii is an anti-inflammatory commensal bacterium identified by gut microbiota analysis of Crohn disease patients. Proc Natl Acad Sci U S A 2008;105:16731–6.

99. Willing B, Halfvarson J, Dicksved J, et al. Twin studies reveal specific imbalances in the mucosa-associated microbiota of patients with ileal Crohn's disease. Inflamm Bowel Dis 2009;15:653–60.

100. Mondot S, Kang S, Furet JP, et al. Highlighting new phylogenetic specificities of Crohn's disease microbiota. Inflamm Bowel Dis 2011;17:185–92.

101. Schwiertz A, Jacobi M, Frick JS, et al. Microbiota in pediatric inflammatory bowel disease. J Pediatr 2010;157:240–4.

102. Garrett WS, Lord GM, Punit S, et al. Communicable ulcerative colitis induced by T-bet deficiency in the innate immune system. Cell 2007;131:33–45.

103. Vijay-Kumar M, Aitken JD, Carvalho FA, et al. Metabolic syndrome and altered gut microbiota in mice lacking Toll-like receptor 5. Science 2010;328:228–31.
104. Borody TJ, Warren EF, Leis SM, et al. Bacteriotherapy using fecal flora: toying with human motions. J Clin Gastroenterol 2004;38:475–83.
105. Grehan MJ, Borody TJ, Leis SM, et al. Durable alteration of the colonic microbiota by the administration of donor fecal flora. J Clin Gastroenterol 2010;44: 551–61.
106. You DM, Franzos MA, Holman RP. Successful treatment of fulminant Clostridium difficile infection with fecal bacteriotherapy. Ann Intern Med 2008;148:632–3.
107. Saavedra JM. Use of probiotics in pediatrics: rationale, mechanisms of action, and practical aspects. Nutr Clin Pract 2007;22:351–65.
108. Ianitti PJ, Palmieri B. Therapeutical use of probiotic formulations in clinical practice. Clin Nutr 2010;29:701–25.

Treatment of Necrotizing Enterocolitis with Probiotics

Kriston Ganguli, MD*, W. Allan Walker, MD

KEYWORDS

- Necrotizing enterocolitis • Preterm infants • Intestinal immunity • Microbiota
- Probiotics

KEY POINTS

- Necrotizing enterocolitis (NEC) is a devastating disease characterized by diffuse intestinal inflammation and necrosis, with few effective preventive and therapeutic options.
- The primary risk factors for the development of NEC are prematurity, immature intestinal immune responses, and bacterial colonization.
- Several functional characteristics of the immature intestine render the preterm infant ill-equipped to manage extrauterine bacterial stimulation.
- Through complex mechanisms, probiotic bacteria modify innate immune responses of the immature intestine, suggesting an effective preventive strategy against NEC.
- Clinical trials demonstrate effectiveness of probiotics in reducing the incidence of NEC as well as data to support the safety of this practice.

Necrotizing enterocolitis (NEC) is the most common gastrointestinal emergency in preterm infants, manifesting as diffuse inflammation and necrosis of the intestine, and is associated with significant morbidity and mortality, as high as 45%.[1] The mean prevalence of NEC in very low birth weight (VLBW) neonates (500–1500 g at birth) in North America is approximately 7% to 12% and occurs in 1% to 5% of infants in the neonatal intensive care unit (NICU).[2,3] The propensity for development of this disease is strongly associated with prematurity and low birth weight, making neonates less than 28 weeks gestation and those with birth weight less than 1000 g the most susceptible population.[4]

The pathogenesis of disease is complex and therefore an active area of research. A critical interplay between bacterial colonization during enteral nutrition initiation and hypoxia-related injury, occurring in a susceptible host, results in an inappropriate,

Conflict of interest: None.
Mucosal Immunology Laboratory, Division of Pediatric Gastroenterology, Massachusetts General Hospital for Children, Harvard Medical School, 114 16th Street, Charlestown, MA 02129-4404, USA
* Corresponding author.
E-mail address: kganguli@partners.org

Gastroenterol Clin N Am 41 (2012) 733–746
http://dx.doi.org/10.1016/j.gtc.2012.08.004
0889-8553/12/$ – see front matter © 2012 Elsevier Inc. All rights reserved.

exaggerated inflammatory response and subsequent intestinal necrosis.[5] Maturity of intestinal innate immune response is directly related to gestational age, placing the preterm infant at an increased risk for development of disease. However, not all premature infants develop NEC, suggesting specific susceptibility beyond gestational age and birth weight. Several additional risk factors have been described, including mode of delivery, source of nutrition, NICU environment, and early exposure to antibiotics.[6] As the process of bacterial colonization is required for the development of NEC, delaying enteral nutrition initiation has been attempted using prolonged parenteral nutrition protocols. This approach may promote intestinal atrophy and compromise feeding success later and has increased risks of infection and prolonged hospitalizations.[7]

If the development of NEC was strictly related to intestinal immune immaturity, one would expect disease development to be solely related to gestational age; however, disease presentation is typically between 7 and 14 days after delivery, regardless of gestational age at birth. This timeline parallels the one required for colonization with anaerobes. Close clinical monitoring is critical during feed initiation, because the signs of developing intestinal inflammation and necrosis may be nonspecific and may progress rapidly. The classic triad at presentation includes (1) feeding intolerance, such as increased gastric residuals or bilious gastric drainage, (2) abdominal distention, and (3) bloody stools. Intestinal perforation, pneumatosis intestinalis, portal venous gas, peritonitis, and hemodynamic instability are signs of severe, rapidly progressing disease and are poor prognostic factors. In addition to the using of abdominal plain radiographs, abdominal sonography may be useful in detecting earlier signs of developing disease, such as increased bowel wall echogenicity and thickness as well as early perfusion compromise.[8,9]

Whether a patient requires medical or surgical management depends on several factors including the severity of disease at presentation and underlying comorbidities, such as baseline ventilatory requirements and cardiovascular status. Most patients respond to medical management (ie, bowel decompression, intravenous hydration, broad-spectrum antibiotics, electrolyte repletion), whereas approximately 30% require urgent surgical resection of necrotic bowel. Infants who survive are at risk for stricture development and those requiring surgical intervention face long-term complications related to short-bowel syndrome, including malabsorption, hyperalimentation dependence, and cholestatic liver disease. In addition to intestinal morbidity, neonates who develop NEC have an increased risk of long-term neurodevelopmental complications, particularly those with severe disease, extremely low birth weight (<1000 g), and associated late bacteremia.[10–12]

In addition to nearly $1 billion in annual expenses required for the acute care of NEC patients in the United States, $1.5 million for every 5 years of ongoing outpatient care of survivors is necessary for management of chronic morbidities.[2,13] Given the aggressive nature of this disease and suboptimal therapeutic options, the clinical focus has appropriately turned to preventive strategies. Currently, breast milk is emphasized as an effective preventive approach in this vulnerable population. In addition to increased concentrations of protective oligosaccharides in breast milk, particularly in the first 15 to 20 weeks of life,[14] stools of infants who are fed breast milk have a significantly higher concentration of lactic acid and lower pH ($P<.05$), compared with formula-fed infants.[15] Although a meta-analysis by McGuire and colleagues[14] demonstrated the protective effects of breast milk against the development of NEC, providing breast milk to all preterm infants is extremely difficult to accomplish in the United States, without an established breast milk banking system. Proposing additional preventive strategies, such as probiotic bacteria, requires an understanding of the multiple complexities, which place preterm infants at risk for developing NEC.

ITY IN PRETERM INFANTS

ınate intestinal immune system renders the premature infant who is
:o manage the immunologic challenges of extrauterine life. The
ıfore delivery is T_H2-predominant and allows avoidance of maternal
ıs. The process of postnatal tolerance is dependent on a transition
ıant to T_H1-predominant immunity and is influenced by the intestinal
The initial stages of bacterial colonization, occurring during the
y and initiation of enteral nutrition, modify intestinal immunity and
f further microbial stimulation.[18,19] Specifically, the interaction
and early colonizing bacteria influences T-lymphocyte development
Recognition of luminal bacterial components by T-lymphocytes is
ce between tolerance and development of gastrointestinal illness.[21]
ıestinal innate immune responses occurs in a predictable manner in
ıowever, this process is poorly regulated in the setting of prematu-
ı immature intestine shows an exaggerated inflammatory response
ıacteria and bacterial products, compared with the mature intestine.
a chemokine, which has the ability to recruit neutrophils to areas of
therefore plays a critical role in the inflammatory response.[22]
I colleagues[23] illustrated a significantly higher expression of IL-8
mRNA) in fetal intestinal epithelium ($P<.05$) and NEC epithelium
ative reverse transcriptase polymerase chain reaction (qRT-PCR),
intestinal epithelium in children older than 1 year (**Fig. 1**A). Nuclear
ıclear factor kappa B (NF-κB) also plays a role in the intestinal
ɔnse. Under the inactivated state, cytosolic NF-κB is bound to inhib-
hich undergoes phosphorylation, ubiquitination, and proteasomal
activated by a proinflammatory stimulus. The ultimate degradation
ıar translocation of NF-κB and subsequent transcription of proin-
ıes. An exaggerated response of this pathway has been demon-
ıature intestine when exposed to colonizing bacteria and may be
ısed expression of IκB in the resting state in immature human enter-
ompared with mature enterocytes (T84 cells).[24] Furthermore, intes-
ɔtor (TLR) activation is downregulated with advancing gestational
contribute to the inflammatory responsiveness in the premature
ıd C show the balance of positive (eg, TLRs, NF-κB) and negative
ɔllip) regulators, which promote a controlled inflammatory
ɔignificant increase in positive inflammatory regulator expression
ırease in negative inflammatory regulator expression ($P<.01$) have
ɔd in fetal intestinal epithelium, compared with mature intestinal
r decreases in negative regulator expression were demonstrated
ithelium from patients with NEC ($P<.001$).[23]
ıct functional characteristics of the preterm intestine, which are
ɾauterine life and sterile amniotic fluid exposure but, however, inap-

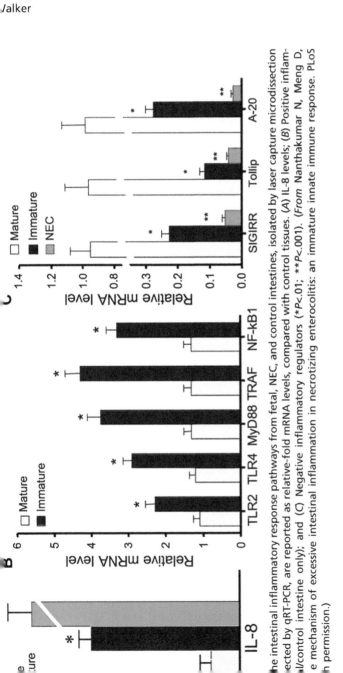

C

Relative mRNA level

1.4
1.2
1.0
0.8
0.3
0.2
0.1
0.0

□ Mature
■ Immature
▨ NEC

SIGIRR   Tollip   A-20

B

Relative mRNA level

6
5
4
3
2
1
0

□ Mature
■ Immature

TLR2 TLR4 MyD88 TRAF NF-kB1

IL-8

he intestinal inflammatory response pathways from fetal, NEC, and control intestines, isolated by laser capture microdissection ected by qRT-PCR, are reported as relative-fold mRNA levels, compared with control tissues. (A) IL-8 levels; (B) Positive inflam-al/control intestine only); and (C) Negative inflammatory regulators (*P<.01; **P<.001). (From Nanthakumar N, Meng D, e mechanism of excessive intestinal inflammation in necrotizing enterocolitis: an immature innate immune response. PLoS n permission.)

ZATION OF PRETERM INFANTS

 at the time of birth is colonized by several bacterial strains and
nvironmental exposures. This process is also affected by several
 factors. The temporal patterns of bacterial acquisition and, ulti-
train diversity are both relatively predictable depending on the
irth, mode of delivery, antibiotic exposure, and source of nutrition.
.l strains include *Bifidobacterium*, *Lactobacillus*, *Escherichia coli*
lostridia, *Staphylococcus*, and *Pseudomonas aeruginosa*.[32] Vagi-
borns are colonized earlier with beneficial strains, such as *Bifido-*
actobacillus, and have smaller populations of *Klebsiella*,
:lostridia, compared with those delivered via cesarean section.[27,32]
terium is the primary colonizing strain of breastfed infants, those
e primarily colonized with *Bifidobacterium* and Bacteroides.[27,33,34]
biome shifts toward that of an adult after completion of weaning.
ocess of preterm infants is further altered by multiple exposures
 the NICU environment, including broad-spectrum antibiotics,
stric acid blockade, and opioids, which compromise intestinal
icated relationship between the various colonizing bacterial strains
al to host health than the presence or absence of one particular
 balance of bacterial diversity promotes intestinal health by
/, decreasing gas production, inhibiting colonization by pathogenic
ving nutrient metabolism and absorption.[6]
sence of luminal bacteria is required in the development of NEC,
ss is considered as an inappropriate inflammatory response to
nts than a bacterial infection.[27] Stool culture analyses during
ave failed to identify a specific organism implicated in the patho-
 Using these techniques, an association has been demonstrated
iella pneumoniae, *Clostridium*, and Enterobacteriaceae.[35–38]
es of stool had previously demonstrated a significant reduction
y and increased density of atypical strains in preterm infants who
ompared with healthy preterm infants.[39,40] Using 16S ribosomal
chniques, Mai and colleagues[41] compared the fecal microbiota
rth weight less than or equal to 1250 g and those younger than
estational ages who developed NEC (Bell Stage ≥II) with matched
ples were analyzed 1 week and 72 hours before the development
ese data showed no statistically significant differences in bacterial
me points in NEC infants or controls, a greater overall variation was
s 1 week before the development of NEC, compared with controls.
s showed a predominance of 4 phyla, Firmicutes, Proteobacteria,
Actinobacteria, with less Actinobacteria and Bacteroidetes in the
ermore, although the 4 predominant phyla were stable between
Proteobacteria increased by 34% and Firmicutes decreased by

Root; bacteria; firmicutes (34.66%)
Root; bacteria; proteobacteria (57.48%)

Root; bacteria; actinobacteria (0.18%)
Root; bacteria; bacteroidetes (0.09%)
Root; bacteria; firmicutes (28.79%)
Root; bacteria; others (0.00%)
Root; bacteria; proteobacteria (70.90%)
Root; bacteria; tennericutes (0.03%)

Cases, <72h of diagnosis

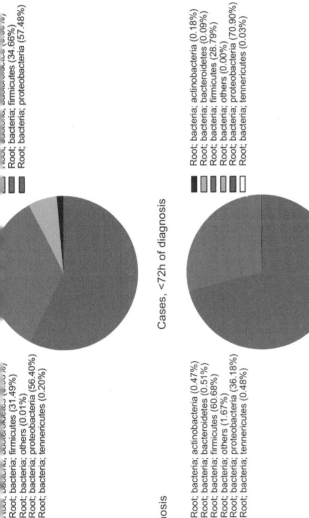
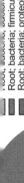

Root; bacteria; firmicutes (31.49%)
Root; bacteria; others (0.01%)
Root; bacteria; proteobacteria (56.40%)
Root; bacteria; tennericutes (0.20%)

eek before diagnosis

Root; bacteria; actinobacteria (0.47%)
Root; bacteria; bacteroidetes (0.51%)
Root; bacteria; firmicutes (60.68%)
Root; bacteria; others (1.67%)
Root; bacteria; proteobacteria (36.18%)
Root; bacteria; tennericutes (0.48%)

of the 4 predominant phyla in 9 patients with NEC, 1 week before and within 72 hours of diagnosis, compared with 9 controls.
, Ukhanova M, et al. Fecal microbiota in premature infants prior to necrotizing enterocolitis. PLoS One 2011;6:e20647; with

composition, intestinal perfusion, and intestinal inflammatory responses.[18,27,44,45] These bacterial effects are compromised in the context of decreased microbiome diversity and increased colonization of pathogenic strains and may play a role in the development of NEC.[2,42,46] Hence, influencing the process of bacterial colonization in the preterm infant, in a favorable way, may be an effective approach to NEC prevention.

The ability of probiotic bacteria to survive intestinal transit, colonize the distal intestinal tract, and exert direct beneficial effects to the host, makes them an optimal strategy in bacterial colonization modulation of the preterm infant. Probiotic strain specificity has been demonstrated, and therefore, choosing optimal strains or strain combinations is necessary when investigating desired immunologic effects. Although our scientific understanding of how probiotic bacteria promote intestinal health is rapidly expanding, the specific mechanism by which probiotics may protect NEC are only partially understood.[47–49] Several experimental models have been used to investigate the mechanisms by which probiotics promote intestinal health and attenuate the exaggerated inflammatory response, characteristic of the immature intestine. Probiotics have been shown to inhibit TLR4 activation, block IκB degradation, activate the antiinflammatory TLR9 protein family, and downregulate IL-6 and tumor necrosis factor α expression in animal models (**Fig. 3**).[50–52]

Several clinical trials have demonstrated a protective effect of orally administered probiotics against the development of NEC in preterm infants. A 2008 Cochrane Collaboration Review of 16 randomized or quasi-randomized controlled trials was published, investigating the use of probiotics in preventing NEC in 2842 preterm infants. Only trials that enrolled infants less than 37 weeks gestational age and/or with birth weight less than 2500 g, and evaluated orally administered probiotics, were included in the review.[53] Each study assessed at least one of the following outcome measures: severe NEC using Bell's criteria (stage II–III), positive blood or cerebral spinal fluid cultures after 5 days of life. Heterogeneity in enrollment criteria,

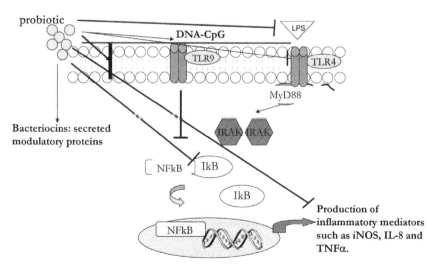

Fig. 3. Several components of the intestinal inflammatory response, which are modified by probiotics in experimental models. (*From* Caplan MS. Probiotics and necrotizing enterocolitis: what have we learned from animal models? Functional Food Reviews 2011;3(1):3–11; with permission.)

control of confounding variables, probiotic regimens, and feeding schedules was noted. In addition, there were limited data to draw conclusions in the extremely low birth weight (ELBW) population. A significant reduction in the incidence of severe NEC (stage ≥II) in probiotic-treated neonates, regardless of birth weight, was demonstrated in 13 studies (relative risk [RR]: 0.35; 95% confidence interval [CI], 0.24–0.52; number needed to treat [NNT[25) and in probiotic-treated neonates with birth weight less than 1500 g in 12 studies (RR: 0.34; 95% CI, 0.23–0.50).

Analysis of 10 studies reporting all-cause mortality showed a significant reduction in probiotic-treated neonates (RR: 0.40; 95% CI, 0.27–0.60), whereas 5 studies that included NEC-associated mortality as an outcome measure showed a significant incidence reduction in the probiotic-treated groups (RR: 0.31; 95% CI, 0.10–0.94). There was no difference in sepsis rates between groups in the 13 trials reporting this measure (RR: 0.90; 95% CI, 0.76–1.07). According to a Cochrane Collaboration methodological quality measure, 4 of the included trials were considered superior and showed a significant reduction in the incidence of NEC in probiotic-treated neonates, compared with controls (RR: 0.25; 95% CI, 0.13–0.49). With the exception of the ELBW population, the data supported the use of probiotics in the prevention of NEC.[53]

In addition, a prospective, double-blind, randomized, controlled clinical trial by Braga and colleagues[54] since the Cochrane Review showed a reduction in the incidence of severe NEC (stage ≥II) in preterm infants between 750 and 1499 g at birth, receiving *B.breve*- or *L.casei*-supplemented human milk, compared with those receiving human milk alone ($P = .05$). Of note, no significant differences in sepsis or mortality risk were demonstrated between groups.

The most recent meta-analysis, by Deshpande and colleagues,[55] in 2010 reviewed 11 randomized controlled trials investigating the effect of an orally administered probiotic regimen on the incidence of severe NEC (stage II–III) in VLBW neonates (<34 weeks gestation and birth weight <1500 g). The trials were conducted between 1997 and 2009, registered in the Cochrane Central database, and included 2176 neonates. The incidence of severe NEC was 6.56% in the control group compared with 2.37% in the probiotic group. A decreased risk of severe NEC was demonstrated in neonates receiving probiotic supplementation, using a fixed-effects analysis (RR: 0.35;95% CI, 0.23–0.55; $P<.00001$ (**Fig. 4**). Minimal heterogeneity was noted between trials, and the NNT was 25 (95% CI: 17,34). Nine of the eleven trials reported all cause mortality and showed a reduced risk in the probiotic-treated neonates compared with controls, again with minimal trial heterogeneity (RR: 0.42; 95% CI, 0.29–0.62; $P<.00001$; NNT 20; 95% CI: 14,34) **Fig. 5**. There was neither significant difference in the incidence of sepsis between groups nor were there significant adverse reported.[1,55]

CONCERNS

Because of several immunologic immaturities, including decreased intestinal barrier integrity, in preterm infants, demonstration of safety in this population is critical. Several well-designed trials have evaluated sepsis and mortality in probiotic-treated preterm infants. Both the meta-analysis in 2010[55] and the Cochrane Review[53] in 2008 concluded that despite heterogeneity in probiotic regimens, there was no increased incidence in outcome measure in probiotic-treated neonates, and no cases of probiotic-related sepsis were reported. However, probiotic-related sepsis has been reported in neonates and other immunocompromised populations previously.[53,55–60] In addition, an increased incidence of sepsis was noted in probiotic-treated neonates in Lin and colleagues's[61] randomized controlled trial. This risk was especially noted in

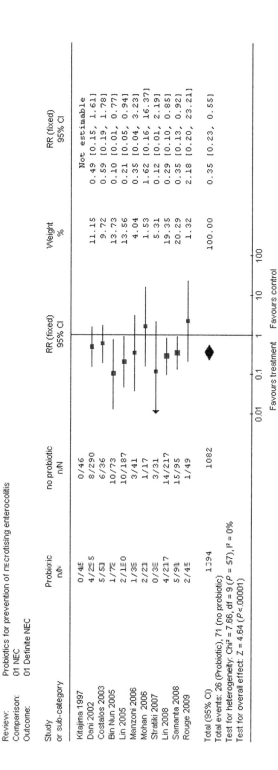

Fig. 4. Probiotics reduce the risk of necrotizing enterocolitis (NEC). (*From* Deshpande G, Roa S, Patole S. Probiotics for preventing necrotizing enterocolitis in preterm neonates: a meta-analysis perspective. Functional Food Reviews 2011;3(1):22–30; with permission.)

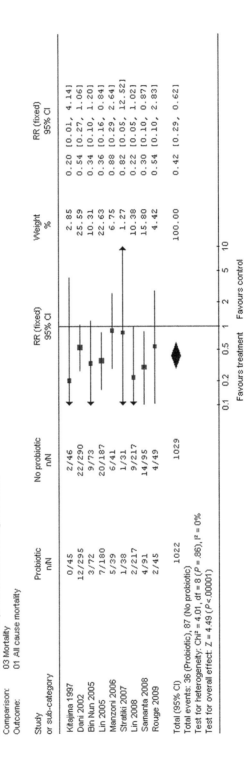

Fig. 5. Probiotics reduce the risk of all-cause mortality. (*From* Deshpande G, Roa S, Patole S. Probiotics for preventing necrotizing enterocolitis in preterm neonates: a meta-analysis perspective. Functional Food Reviews 2011;3(1):22–30; with permission.)

the population of neonates with less than 750 g birth weight and, none of the septic patients grew Lactobacillus or Bifidobacterium spp. on blood culture.

Recent data, using human in vitro models of NEC, have demonstrated the ability of intact components or secreted factors of probiotic bacteria to attenuate the LPS and IL-1-β–induced intestinal inflammatory response (unpublished data). This is an area of active investigation, as these bacteria-free factors may offer an effective preventive approach without bacteria-associated safety concerns.

SUMMARY

The primary risk factor for the development of NEC is prematurity. Intestinal function and innate intestinal immunity of the fetus promote growth and survival in the sterile intrauterine environment and mature with advancing gestational age. At term, the intestine is equipped to manage the drastic changes and multiple microbial challenges of extrauterine life. When a neonate is born premature, the inevitable interaction between the immature intestine and luminal bacteria results in an exaggerated inflammatory response, progressing to the diffuse inflammation and necrosis of NEC, in a susceptible host. The process of bacterial colonization in the premature infant is negatively altered by several environmental factors and results in a less beneficial microbiota balance and variety.

Probiotic bacteria may alter the intestinal microbiome in an advantageous way, promoting a more mature microbial profile. A statistically significant reduction in the incidence of NEC in preterm infants receiving orally administered probiotics has been demonstrated in multiple randomized controlled trials. Because of trial design heterogeneity, optimal strain, dose, timing of administration, and host characteristics have not been determined. Although strain-specific immunologic effects have been demonstrated using in vitro NEC models, the decreased incidence of NEC in various heterogeneous trials suggests an effect that may be less strain specific in clinical application. Although a rigorous review of previously conducted clinical trials for safety concerns has been reassuring, the relative immaturities of preterm infants make this a particularly vulnerable population.

Although the care of premature infants continues to advance, minimal improvements have been made in the prevention and management of necrotizing enterocolitis. Ongoing investigation using in vitro models, with a particular focus on mechanisms to explain the antiinflammatory properties of probiotic bacteria, is critical. These data will allow more sophisticated clinical application in the future and would offer a basis with which a single protocol clinical trial could be designed, investigating the use of probiotics in the prevention of NEC. Current clinical trial data are promising; however, repeated multicenter clinical investigation using a single protocol is required to ensure reproducibility, safety, and efficacy. This investigation would allow the scientific and medical communities the necessary confidence to support routine clinical use of probiotics in the prevention of this devastating disease in preterm infants.

REFERENCES

1. Deshpande G, Roa S, Patole S. Probiotics for preventing necrotizing enterocolitis in preterm neonates: a meta-analysis perspective. Functional Food Reviews 2011;3:22–30.
2. Neu J, Walker WA. Necrotizing Enterocolitis. N Engl J Med 2011;364:255–64.
3. Holman RC, Stoll BJ, Curns AT, et al. Necrotising enterocolitis hospitalisations among neonates in the United States. Paediatr Perinat Epidemiol 2006;20: 498–506.

4. Rowe MI, Reblock KK, Kurkchubasche AG, et al. Necrotizing enterocolitis in the extremely low birth weight infant. J Pediatr Surg 1994;29:987–90.

5. Hsueh W, Caplan MS, Qu XW, et al. Neonatal necrotizing enterocolitis: clinical considerations and pathogenetic concepts. Pediatr Dev Pathol 2003;6:6–23.

6. Ganguli K, Walker WA. Probiotics in the prevention of necrotizing enterocolitis. J Clin Gastroenterol 2011;45(Suppl):S133–8.

7. Stoll BJ, Hansen N, Fanaroff AA, et al. Late-onset sepsis in very low birth weight neonates: the experience of the NICHD Neonatal Research Network. Pediatrics 2002;110:285–91.

8. Epelman M, Daneman A, Navarro OM, et al. Necrotizing enterocolitis: review of state-of-the-art imaging findings with pathologic correlation. Radiographics 2007;27:285–305.

9. Faingold R, Daneman A, Tomlinson G, et al. Necrotizing enterocolitis: assessment of bowel viability with color Doppler US. Radiology 2005;235:587–94.

10. Lin PW, Stoll BJ. Necrotising enterocolitis. Lancet 2006;368:1271–83.

11. Schulzke SM, Desphande GC, Patole SK. Neurodevelopmental outcome of very low birth weight infants with necrotizing enterocolitis-a systematic review of observational studies. Arch Pediatr Adolesc Med 2007;161:583–90.

12. Martin CR, Dammann O, Allred EN, et al. Neurodevelopment of extremely preterm infants who had necrotizing enterocolitis with or without late bacteremia. J Pediatr 2010;157:751–756.e1.

13. Spencer AU, Kocevich D, McKinney-Barnett M, et al. Pediatric short-bowel syndrome: the cost of comprehensive care. Am J Clin Nutr 2008;88:1552–9.

14. McGuire W, Anthony MY. Formula milk versus preterm human milk in preterm or LBW infants (cochrane review). Cochrane Database Syst Rev 2001;(3):CD002972.

15. Ogawa K, Ben RA, Pons S, et al. Volatile fatty acids, lactic acid, and pH in the stools of breast-fed and bottle-fed infants. J Pediatr Gastroenterol Nutr 1992; 15:248–52.

16. Salzman N, Underwood M, Bevins C. Paneth cells, defensins, and the commensal microbiota: a hypothesis on intimate interplay at the intestinal mucosa. Semin Immunol 2007;19:70–83.

17. Morein B, Blomquist G, Hu K. Immune responsiveness in the neonatal period. J Comp Pathol 2007;137(Suppl 1):S27–31.

18. Otte JM, Podolsky DK. Functional modulation of enterocytes by gram-positive and gram-negative microorganisms. Am J Physiol Gastrointest Liver Physiol 2004;286:G613–26.

19. Abreu MT. The Ying and yang of bacterial signaling in necrotizing enterocolitis. Gastroenterology 2010;138:39–43.

20. Rosenfeldt V, Michaelsen KF, Jakobsen M, et al. Effect of probiotic Lactobacillus strains in young children hospitalized with acute diarrhea. Pediatr Infect Dis J 2002;21:411–6.

21. Thomas DW, Greer FR, American Academy of Pediatrics Committee on Nutrition, et al. Probiotics and prebiotics in pediatrics. Pediatrics 2010;126:1217–31.

22. Huber AR, Kunkel SL, Todd RF, et al. Regulation of transendothelial neutrophil migration by endogenous interleukin-8. Science 1991;254:99–102.

23. Nanthakumar N, Meng D, Goldstein AM, et al. The mechanism of excessive intestinal inflammation in necrotizing enterocolitis: an immature innate immune response. PLoS One 2011;6:e17776.

24. Claud EC, Lu L, Anton PM, et al. Developmentally regulated IkappaB expression in intestinal epithelium and susceptibility to flagellin-induced inflammation. Proc Natl Acad Sci U S A 2004;101:7404–8.

25. Fusunyan RD, Nanthakumar NN, Baldeon ME, et al. Evidence for an innate immune response in the immature intestine: toll-like receptors on fetal enterocytes. Pediatr Res 2001;49:589–93.
26. Liew FY, Xu D, Brint EK, et al. Negative regulation of toll-like receptor-mediated immune responses. Nat Rev Immunol 2005;5:446–58.
27. Claud EC. Bacterial colonization of the preterm infant gut: unique susceptibilities and neonatal necrotizing enterocolitis. Functional Food Reviews 2011;3(1):12–21.
28. Dai D, Nanthakumar NN, Newburg DS, et al. Role of oligosaccharides and glycoconjugates in intestinal host defense. J Pediatr Gastroenterol Nutr 2000;30: S23–33.
29. Lin J, Holzman IR, Jiang P, et al. Expression of intestinal trefoil factor in developing rat intestine. Biol Neonate 1999;76:92–7.
30. Salzman NH, Polin RA, Harris MC, et al. Enteric defensin expression in necrotizing enterocolitis. Pediatr Res 1998;44:20–6.
31. Snyder JD, Walker WA. Structure and function of intestinal mucin: developmental aspects. Int Arch Allergy Appl Immunol 1987;82:351–6.
32. Claud EC, Walker WA. Bacterial colonization, probiotics, and necrotizing enterocolitis. J Clin Gastroenterol 2008;42:S46–52.
33. Conroy M, Shi HN, Walker WA. The long-term health effects of neonatal microbial flora. Curr Opin Allergy Clin Immunol 2009;9:197–201.
34. Harmsen HJ, Wildeboer-Veloo AC, Raangs GC, et al. Analysis of intestinal flora development in breast-fed and formula-fed infants by using molecular identification and detection methods. J Pediatr Gastroenterol Nutr 2000;30:61–7.
35. Bell MH, Feigen RD, Ternberg JL. Changes in the incidence of necrotizing enterocolitis associated with variation of the gastrointestinal microflora in neonates. Am J Surg 1979;138:629–31.
36. Millar MR, MacKay P, Levene M, et al. *Enterobacteriaceae* and neonatal necrotising enterocolitis. Arch Dis Child 1992;67(1 Spec No):53–6.
37. Sturm R, Staneck JL, Stauffer LR, et al. Neonatal necrotizing enterocolitis associated with penicillin-resistant, toxigenic *Clostridium butyricum*. Pediatrics 1980;66: 928–31.
38. Bell MJ, Shackelford P, Feigin RD, et al. Epidemiologic and bacteriologic evaluation of neonatal necrotizing enterocolitis. J Pediatr Surg 1979;14:1–4.
39. Wang Y, Hoenig JD, Malin KJ, et al. 16s rRNA gene-based analysis of fecal microbiota from preterm infants with and without necrotizing enterocolitis. ISME J 2009; 3:944–54.
40. Mshvildadze M, Neu J, Shuster J, et al. Intestinal microbial ecology in premature infants assessed with non-culture-based techniques. J Pediatr 2010;156:20–5.
41. Mai V, Young CM, Ukhanova M, et al. Fecal microbiota in premature infants prior to necrotizing enterocolitis. PLoS One 2011;6:e20647.
42. Claud EC, Walker WA. Hypothesis: inappropriate colonization of the premature intestine can cause neonatal necrotizing enterocolitis. FASEB J 2001;15: 1398–403.
43. Morowitz MJ, Poroyko V, Caplan M, et al. Redefining the role of intestinal microbes in the pathogenesis of necrotizing enterocolitis. Pediatrics 2010;125: 777–85.
44. Hooper LV, Wong MH, Thelin A, et al. Molecular analysis of commensal host-microbial relationships in the intestine. Science 2001;291:881–4.
45. Mack DR, Michail S, Wei S, et al. Probiotics inhibit enteropathogenic *E. coli* adherence in vitro by inducing intestinal mucin gene expression. Am J Physiol 1999; 276(4 Pt 1):G941–50.

46. Gareau MG, Sherman PM, Walker WA. Probiotics and the gut microbiota in intestinal health and disease. Nat Rev Gastroenterol Hepatol 2010;7:503–14.

47. Foligne B, Nutten S, Grangette C, et al. Correlation between in vitro and in vivo immunomodulatory properties of lactic acid bacteria. World J Gastroenterol 2007;13:236–43.

48. He F, Morita H, Hashimoto H, et al. Intestinal *bifidobacterium* species induce varying cytokine production. J Allergy Clin Immunol 2002;109:1035–6.

49. Khailova L, Dvorak K, Arganbright KM, et al. *Bifidobacterium bifidum* improves intestinal integrity in a rat model of necrotizing enterocolitis. Am J Physiol Gastrointest Liver Physiol 2009;297:G940–9.

50. Caplan MS. Probiotics and necrotizing enterocolitis: what have we learned from animal models? Functional Food Reviews 2011;3:3–11.

51. Neish AS, Gewitz AT, Zeng H, et al. Prokaryotic regulation of epithelial responses by inhibition of IkappaB-alpha ubiquitination. Science 2000;289:1560–3.

52. Chen CC, Louie S, Shi HN, et al. Preinoculation with the probiotic *Lactobacillus acidophilus* early in life effectively inhibits murine *Citrobacter rodentium* colitis. Pediatr Res 2005;58:1185–91.

53. Alfaleh K, Anabrees J, Bassler D, et al. Probiotics for prevention of necrotizing enterocolitis in preterm infants. Cochrane Database Syst Rev 2011;(3):CD005496.

54. Braga TD, da Silva GA, de Lira PI, et al. Efficacy of *Bifidobacterium breve* and *Lactobacillus casei* oral supplementation on necrotizing enterocolitis in very-low-birth-weight preterm infants: a double-blind, randomized, controlled trial. Am J Clin Nutr 2011;93:81–6.

55. Deshpande G, Rao S, Patole S, et al. Updated meta-analysis of probiotics for preventing necrotizing enterocolitis in preterm neonates. Pediatrics 2010;125: 921–30.

56. Thompson C, McCarter YS, Krause PJ, et al. *Lactobacillus acidophilus* sepsis in a neonate. J Perinatol 2001;21:258–60.

57. Broughton RA, Gruber WC, Haffar AA, et al. Neonatal meningitis due to *lactobacillus*. Pediatr Infect Dis 1983;2:382–4.

58. Perapoch J, Planes AM, Querol A, et al. Fungemia with *Saccharomyces cerevisiae* in two newborns, only one of whom had been treated with ultra-levure. Eur J Clin Microbiol Infect Dis 2000;19:468–70.

59. Ohishi A, Takahashi S, Ito Y, et al. *Bifidobacterium* septicemia associated with postoperative probiotic therapy in a neonate with omphalocele. J Pediatr 2010; 156:679–81.

60. Land MH, Rouster-Stevens K, Woods CR, et al. *Lactobacillus* sepsis associated with probiotic therapy. Pediatrics 2005;115:178–81.

61. Lin HC, Hsu CH, Chen HL. Oral probiotics prevent necrotizing enterocolitis in very low birth weight preterm infants: a multicenter, randomized, controlled trial. Pediatrics 2008;122:693–700.

Probiotics in the Development and Treatment of Allergic Disease

Erika Isolauri, MD, PhD[a],*, Samuli Rautava, MD, PhD[a],
Seppo Salminen, PhD[b]

KEYWORDS

• Allergy • Breastfeeding • Immunology • Infant • Nutrition • Pregnancy • Probiotics

KEY POINTS

- Allergic diseases constitute the most common chronic diseases of childhood.
- Early nutrition exerts short- and long-term effects on health of the host by programming its immunologic, metabolic, and microbiologic development.
- Recent scientific advances demonstrate that deviations in gut microbiota composition precede development of the allergic phenotype, inviting preventive and therapeutic applications.
- To reverse the increasing burden of allergic diseases, the joint action of specific nutrients and probiotics on the intestinal milieu can be exploited.
- The rationale of probiotic intervention comprises restoration of the properties of the unbalanced indigenous microbiota, control of the inflammatory response, and tolerance induction.
- The clinical benefit depends on host characteristics and properties of probiotic strains, strain combinations, and their interactions with nutritional components in food.

THE HYGIENE HYPOTHESIS AND GUT MICROBIOTA: THE STARTING POINT

The epidemiologic evidence indicating that early exposure to microbes is associated with a reduced risk of developing atopic sensitization and atopic disease is abundant, and the development of allergic diseases has been attributed to reduced microbial contact.[1] People living in affluent hygienic environments lack the pressure of microbial stimulation, in particular the diversity of microbial contact that has evolved between the host and the gut microbiota, the total genetic pool of the microbiome. The same

Disclosures: None.
[a] Department of Paediatrics, University of Turku and Turku University Hospital, Kiinamyllynkatu 4-8, 20520 Turku, Finland; [b] Functional Foods Forum, University of Turku, Itäinen Pitkäkatu 4 A, Turku, Finland
* Corresponding author.
E-mail address: erika.isolauri@utu.fi

progression is seen in human nutrition. A shift in food preservation from drying and natural fermentation to industrial pasteurization and sterilization has reduced the microbial exposure associated with food intake. Moreover, a switch from a low-fat, plant-polysaccharide–rich diet to a high-fat, high-sugar diet, collectively described as the Western diet, immediately alters the microbiota composition in the gastrointestinal tract.[2]

The shift of emphasis in the hygiene hypothesis has thus evolved from acute infection protecting from atopic disease[3,4] to a balanced gut microbiota, the earliest and most massive source of microbial exposure, protecting from the chronic inflammatory conditions, collectively characterized as Western lifestyle diseases.[1] Indeed, environmental changes in the industrialized world reducing microbial contact at an early age have occurred concomitant with the growing epidemic of atopic eczema, allergic rhinoconjunctivitis, and asthma, but also with diseases phenotypically as different as inflammatory bowel disease and type I diabetes, and obesity with its comorbidities.[5–7] All in all, the development of these conditions points to a failure to generate and maintain a balanced host-microbe interaction, resulting in a tolerogenic milieu in the mucosae, the interface between the internal and external environments of the host. Our conception of the microbes has thus changed; traditional thinking links microbes directly to pathogens and so consequently to acute disease, whereas the current view brings to the fore the microbiome as an important organ of host defense operating at the intersection between host genotype and diet to modulate the host's adaptation to the modern environment.

The rationale of probiotic intervention here is to provide safe, timely, and sufficient microbial contact to avert the establishment of a deviant gut microbiota and immune responsiveness, and thereby reduce the risk of immunoinflammatory disease. An aberrant gut microbiota composition may result in delayed maturation of gut barrier function, or the perturbation may follow on environmental triggering (ie, gut microbiota changes may precede the development of chronic disease or be merely a consequence of a local inflammatory response). There are data on record to support both conceptions.

It seems that the compositional development of the gut microbiota differs between infants evincing and not evincing atopic manifestations. Healthy infants harbor a natural predominance of bifidobacteria with specific strains, whereas those later developing atopic disease have more *Clostridium* species and fewer *Bifidobacterium* species in stools compared with nonatopics.[8,9] Allergic infants seem to be colonized mainly with *Bifidobacterium adolescentis*, and healthy infants mainly with *Bifidobacterium bifidum* and *Bifidobacterium longum*. The intestinal *Bifidobacterium* species from allergic infants have been shown to induce proinflammatory cytokine production, in contrast to those from healthy infants,[10] suggesting a need for a more precise characterization at species and strain levels of the healthy gut microbiota. Sequence-based information has recently accumulated, but most of the current methods fail in species or strain-level identification of microbiota components. The precise identification process needs to be completed before the microbial communities can successfully be modulated toward health.[11]

ALLERGIC DISORDERS: A MOVING TARGET FOR THERAPEUTIC AND PREVENTIVE MEASURES?

Allergic disorders represent a profound pediatric health problem, the most common chronic disease state among children. Notwithstanding the extensive scientific interest centered on this problem, research so far has been unable to conclusively ascertain the determinants underlying the epidemic of allergy. However, the most recent advances in research into chronic inflammatory disease have uncovered similarities in the mechanisms of diseases of the T helper (Th) 1-type, such as inflammatory bowel disease, and atopic disease of the Th2-type, and obesity, and thereby opened up new angles on the role of environmental exposures in the development and perpetuation of allergic disease.[12] Specifically, studies on microbial contact early in life, including probiotic research, have linked aberrant gut microbiota and inflammatory responses during critical periods of maturation to perturbed immunologic homeostasis.

Immune priming by microbial exposure may be essential particularly for the gut-associated immune system to fulfill its two opposing functions: mounting a brisk response to pathogens and maintaining hyporesponsiveness to innocuous antigens. The healthy gut microbiota shapes the host responder type and its resilience to environmental offense (reviewed in[1,12]). Recent experimental and clinical reports also highlight the way the immune regulation exerted by the gut microbiota extends to systemic immunity[13] and to peripheral tissues, such as the lung.[14] Current research interest is focused on these active immunologic processes promoting tolerance and their potential for exploitation in clinical intervention studies. However, deeper insight into the multiple mechanisms of allergic disease is still needed for the validation of specific strains carrying antiallergic potential.

Epigenetic variables tie the hereditary susceptibility to the allergic phenotype in general, but not to definite allergic diseases. The heterogeneous manifestations of what are called "allergic disorders" (ie, the diverse phenotypes) remain clinically and immunologically poorly defined, and consequently no universal remedy can be expected. Hence, evaluation of the probiotic potential as an alternative to attain prophylactic or therapeutic effect in "allergic disorders" calls for an accurate characterization of the target: definition of the study population, in terms of age, immune responder type, diet, including the presence or absence of food allergies, and the composition and activity of the existing gut microbiota, exemplifying common determinants interacting with probiotics.

Because of confusion in the definition of allergic disorders, alternative approaches have been endorsed. These include scientific validation of and criteria for markers to support health claims for foods, including probiotics,[15] the current ILSI Europe working group on "Monitoring immune modulation by nutrition in the general population," which focuses on adapting methodology to assess risk reduction in the healthy European consumers.[16,17] In a similar manner, the European Science Foundation has gathered a forward look assessment to cover future research targets in this area.[12]

To define the strategic direction for clinical studies, one hypothesis has been pinpointed as a working target for probiotics in the development and treatment of allergic conditions[18]: impaired barrier functions of the skin epithelium and gut mucosa, including the local microbiota in these functions (**Fig. 1**). Specific probiotics counteract the hypersensitivity process by modifying the immunomodulatory activity of dietary antigens, and potentiate the host's endogenous defense mechanisms by stabilizing the gut mucosal barrier function.

It seems justified to expect that clinical research focusing on the critical window and the mechanisms involved, together with the environmental elements that interact with the most effective probiotic strains, will devise novel preventive therapies.

ESTABLISHMENT OF THE GUT MICROBIOTA: NEW INSIGHT INTO PROBIOTIC ACTION

Environmental exposures during the critical stage of maturation may directly shape the risk of disease. Certain sources of exposure go beyond all others: the establishment of

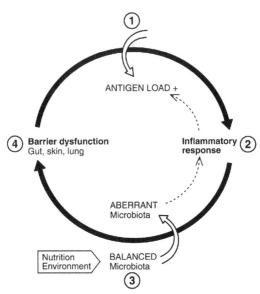

Fig. 1. Targets of probiotic therapy in allergic disease. Different internal and external challenges may trigger inflammatory responses, which may direct the composition and function of gut microbiota to become aberrant and proinflammatory; a strong inflammatory response may be mounted against indigenous bacteria, leading to perpetuation of the inflammation and gut barrier dysfunction. Specific probiotics may counteract the inflammatory process by the following: (1) Promoting the exclusion of antigens, enhancing the degradation of enteral antigens, altering their immunogenicity, and thereby reducing the antigen load. (2) Regulation of the secretion of proinflammatory and anti-inflammatory mediators, and direction of the development of the immune system during the critical period of life when the risk of allergic disease is heightened. (3) Normalization of the properties of unbalanced indigenous microbiota. (4) Normalizing the composition of the intestinal microbiota, normalizing the increased intestinal permeability associated with intestinal inflammation.

the gut microbiota, the mode of delivery, and breastfeeding. Recent experimental and clinical studies have demonstrated that the mother's nutritional status and immune responses during pregnancy, and the mode of delivery and breastfeeding/breast milk composition, all exert an important impact, the gut microbiota interacting with all other elements in the nutritional, immunologic, and microbiologic programming of child health (**Fig. 2**).

Compositional Development of the Gut Microbiota

Although colonization process in the infant gut has been intensively studied, the early events guiding microbiome development remain unresolved. Establishment of the gut microbiota can be characterized by three steps. The first step of colonization at and after birth involves mainly facultative anaerobic bacteria. Among the colonizers are bacteria derived from the mother's gut and skin, including *Escherichia coli*, clostridia, staphylococci, and some *Bacteroides* species.[19]

The second step comprises a rapid succession by anaerobic genera, such as *Bifidobacterium*, *Eubacterium*, *Clostridium*, and increases in *Bacteroides* species, especially in breastfed infants. Different species of bifidobacteria can range from 60% up to 90% of the total fecal microbiota in breastfed infants and frequently the composition

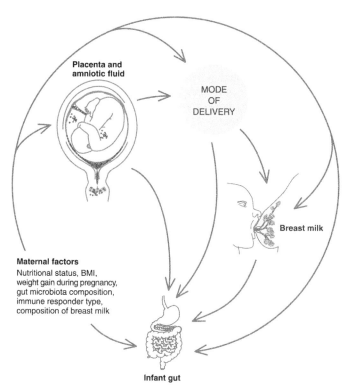

Fig. 2. Microbiologic programming of child health. Targets of probiotic intervention in reducing the risk of allergic disease in early life. The nutritional and immunologic status of the mother during pregnancy and lactation and the mode of delivery all impact on child health influencing the initial compositional development of gut microbiota of the newborn and breast milk composition, with the maternal gut microbiota interacting with all these elements. BMI, body mass index.

comprises *Bifidobacterium breve*, *B infantis*, and *B longum* species, whereas the most common lactobacilli in breastfed and formula-fed infant feces are usually related to the *Lactobacillus acidophilus* group.[19,20]

The third major step coincides with weaning, which heralds a major shift leading to a microbiome consisting of microbial consortia characteristic of the adult microbiota.[21,22] During this step, rapid changes also take place in energy-harvesting *Bacteroides* species, these increasing a thousandfold. The adult type of microbiota has been estimated to be achieved by 2 to 3 years of age.[21] Shifts in abundance in major taxonomic groups occur during this time period, this presumably reflecting the diet or health status of the host.[22]

Microbial Contact in Prenatal, Perinatal, and Postnatal Periods

Current dogma defines fetal life as microbiologically sterile except in cases of infection. Investigations on microbial growth during the fetal period make no reference to the normal microbiota before delivery and the newborn gut has also been described as sterile.[19] The intrauterine environment is likely to be protected from and protective against pathogenics, but it is coming to be accepted that a very selective microbial exposure ensues already before birth, because placenta and amniotic fluid contain specific bacteria.[23,24] Particularly, placenta samples after extremely premature deliveries have been documented to contain diverse bacteria.[25] Conversely, pathogenic bacteria in the placenta and amniotic membranes may lead to premature birth, or to neonatal and maternal infection. However, there are data suggesting that small quantities of microbes are also present in the fetoplacental area in term pregnancies, but their sources and roles remain undefined. One mechanism and route for the exposures currently being investigated is through the maternal mucosal system.[24] The recently reported presence of bacterial DNA in the neonate meconium likewise tends to corroborate the prenatal origin of microbes.[26]

Taken together, one could consider the microbiota transfer from the mother to the newborn during the perinatal period as a continuum and as reflecting the close environment. This inoculum may induce adaptation to the anticipated postnatal environment, concomitantly impacting on later disease susceptibility.

Breastfeeding

After birth, microbial contact continues through breastfeeding. Human milk is generally considered the optimal nutrition for neonates because it contains the required nutrients and protective compounds, including specific oligosaccharides and fatty acids influencing early microbial colonization, but also specific microbiota and molecules operating in host-microbe interaction. Indeed, there is abundant evidence that breast milk also transmits bacteria to the infant gut[27]: the mother provides the infant with bifidobacteria, lactic acid bacteria, and other microbiota components in significant quantities during breastfeeding. Breastfeeding also exposes the infant to the mother's skin bacteria. Perez and colleagues[28] have shown that some bacterial signatures in breast milk are common to the infant's feces and mother's blood samples, which implies a link. Hence, the milk microbiota contains a distinct bacterial community from skin, gut, vagina, or mouth.[29]

The microbiota transfer can constitute a protective microbiota or mediate the mother's aberrant microbiota composition to the infant,[30,31] depending on maternal health and nutritional state. Collado and coworkers[32] have shown that the composition and development of the infant gut microbiota are influenced by the body mass index (BMI), weight, and weight gain of the mother during pregnancy. In a similar manner, mothers with allergic disease have deranged counts of bifidobacteria in breast milk and the maternal fecal and breast-milk bifidobacterial counts guide the compositional development of the *Bifidobacterium* microbiota in the infant.[30]

Mode of Delivery

The mode of delivery has been reported to impact on microbiota transfer from the mother to the infant and the effects are present immediately after birth, but also beyond infancy.[33–35] The mode of delivery has been demonstrated to influence the acquisition and structure of the initial microbiota in multiple body habitats in newborns,[34] especially in respect of the levels of *Clostridium difficile*, which may subsequently influence the risk of atopic manifestations.[36] Moreover, it has recently been demonstrated that the mode of delivery has an impact on breast milk microbial composition, which differs strikingly between mothers delivering vaginally and those undergoing caesarean section, but interestingly also between the type of caesarean delivery (elective vs nonelective caesarean sections).[29] These observations suggest that the lack of physiologic stress or hormonal signals during labor may influence the process of microbial transmission to the mother's milk.

PROBIOTICS: DEFINITIONS AND SPECIFICATIONS

According to the World Health Organization definition probiotics are "Live microorganisms which when administered in adequate amounts confer a health benefit on the host."[37] The definition also requires the use of a nomenclature of bacteria, which conforms to the current, scientifically recognized terminology. Bacteria should be characterized and deposited in international culture collections with deposit numbers to ensure consistency in research. These are the requirements most scientific journals also set forth to facilitate the understanding and interpretation of results concerning specific probiotics. However, other factors hitherto overlooked impacting on probiotic properties include the manufacturing process and the food matrix used. Both have been reported to modify probiotic properties significantly.[38,39] Such interaction should also be assessed before human intervention studies.[38,40]

Strict adherence to the code of strain specifications and identification of manufacturer and probiotic quality and viability measures would also aid in strain-specific meta-analysis and comprehensive reviews on probiotic efficacy. For instance, most nutrition journals require authors to deposit the microbial strains they use in any study submitted in publicly accessible culture collections (eg, the American Type Culture Collection) and to refer to the collection and strain numbers in the text. When the authenticity of subcultures of culture collection specimens that are distributed by individuals cannot be ensured, authors should indicate the relevant laboratory strain designations and donor sources, and the original culture collection identification numbers.

EVIDENCE OF PROBIOTIC ACTION: HOW TO INTERPRET CLINICAL DATA

There are data on record to indicate that the gut microbiota composition can discriminate between allergic and healthy children, and that the distinction may precede the clinical disease. The role of the gut microbiota in allergic disease, and by the same token that of probiotics, may also be assessed indirectly: mode of delivery, breastfeeding, and breast milk composition all impact on the gut microbiota on one hand and on allergic disease on the other,[30,35,41] whereas the gut microbiota composition has a bearing on allergic disease.[8,9]

The effects of probiotics have been attributed to restoration to normal of increased intestinal permeability and unbalanced gut microbiota, improvement of the intestine's immunologic barrier functions, and reduced generation of proinflammatory cytokines characteristic of local and systemic allergic inflammation (see **Fig. 1**). The potential of specific strains of the gut microbiota to contribute to the generation of Th1- and Th3-type immune responses counterregulating the Th2-type immune responses in atopic disease may create optimal conditions to redirect the polarized immunologic memory of the newborn to a healthy balance and thereby reduce the disease risk. This activity may prove an attractive tool in fighting environmental stimuli accompanied by gut barrier dysfunction throughout infancy and early childhood. Modification of the gut microbiota together with immunomodulatory effects may serve to decipher the probiotic potential of specific strains.

Several reports have been published of clinical studies on probiotics in the prevention and treatment of allergic disease. Strikingly, there are currently even more reviews and meta-analyses, but few recommendations. The reason for this could be related to poor characterization of the various probiotic effects or the conditions studied, both of which remain major challenges in the probiotic literature (**Box 1**). In the early reviews, different probiotic strains were simply plotted together despite the fact that each strain and also each combination of strains is unique. Moreover, children with food allergy

> **Box 1**
> **Problems in current probiotic literature**
>
> - Not all members of the healthy gut microbiota can be used as probiotics
> - Only some bifidobacteria or lactobacilli carry probiotic potential, preclinical testing mandatory
> - Each probiotic strain is unique with specific local and systemic immunomodulatory effects and influences on the gut microbiota
> - Effects of probiotic combinations differ from individual probiotics, effects may be additive, or even counteractive
> - Production methods and delivery food matrices impact on probiotic efficacy
> - The probiotic effects depend on the host characteristics (existing gut microbiota, immune responder type, clinical condition, particularly the presence or absence of intestinal involvement, diet, and the immediate environment)

have been compared with those without the intestinal involvement of allergic disease, and demonstration of the different immunologic effects of the food matrix has been neglected. In studies aiming to reduce the risk of atopic disease in populations at high risk, data regarding fundamental variables that may modify disease risk (eg, the precise hereditary risk based on family history or the duration of breastfeeding) have been variably reported and not always taken into account in meta-analyses. Moreover, the route, timing, and duration of probiotic supplementation, all of which have implications for the presumed mechanisms of probiotic action, vary between the published studies. Systematic reviews and meta-analyses may also carry a systematic risk in setting the selection criteria. Obviously, published clinical intervention trials are known to the scientific community and biased selection among them for review multiplies the problem. More recently, the systematic and statistical problems attending repetition of the same meta-analyses have likewise been recognized.[42]

For these reasons, only well-characterized (with definition of the manufacturing processes used) and preclinically tested strains should be applied in clinical intervention studies, together with specification of the population (age, immune responder type, symptoms, presence or absence of challenge-proved food allergies, diet, and existing gut microbiota composition), to target putative mechanisms of the disease.

Probiotics in Prevention of Atopic Disease

To date, results from 11 clinical trials assessing the effects of probiotic intervention in early infancy to reduce the risk of atopic disease have to our knowledge been published (**Table 1**).[43,46–52,54–56] Although probiotic supplementation has not been associated with adverse effects in any study, the results concerning clinical efficacy are conflicting, this possibly resulting from differences in the probiotic strains used, the age at which the intervention commenced, and the duration of the intervention, and confounding factors, such as diet and hereditary risk in the target population. Nonetheless, a meticulous review of the trials published may give important insight into probiotic effects in early life.

Based on currently published data, it may be argued that prenatal maternal supplementation enhances the efficacy of probiotics in reducing the risk of eczema in the infant. The seven trials thus far published[43,47–49,52,54,55] showing the efficacy of early probiotic intervention in reducing the risk of eczema all include prenatal maternal and postnatal probiotic supplementation. In contrast, probiotic supplementation during the prenatal and postnatal periods failed to reduce the risk of eczema in only one study, in a population with prolonged breastfeeding, potentially necessitating distinct power calculation,[50] whereas both of the published trials in which probiotic supplementation was given postnatally directly to the infants revealed no differences between the intervention and placebo groups.[46,51] According to one recent meta-analysis,[57] prenatal maternal probiotic supplementation is effective in reducing eczema risk. However, the trials included in the meta-analysis also included postnatal intervention and in a relatively recent study conducted in Australia, maternal prenatal supplementation with the probiotic *Lactobacillus rhamnosus* GG alone was not sufficient to reduce the occurrence of eczema in the offspring.[56] Collectively, these data suggest that only maternal probiotic intervention during pregnancy and breastfeeding may be effective in reducing the risk of eczema in the infant. In line with this notion, subgroup analysis data suggesting that *L rhamnosus* GG administered to the pregnant and breastfeeding mother significantly reduces the risk of eczema in high-risk infants have been reported.[58]

There are also data suggesting that probiotics may reduce the risk of atopic disease also later in infancy, because supplementation with the probiotic *Lactobacillus* F19 initiated at the time of weaning seems to be effective in reducing the cumulative incidence of eczema in the infant from the development of eczema until the age of 13 months,[53] but whether the effect persists is unclear. In general, the relatively short follow-up periods in the published trials hinder proper assessment of preventive effects and it is therefore of the utmost importance to continue the follow-up of study subjects and report more long-term outcomes. On a conceptual level, the question of what may be considered to constitute a preventive effect may be posed.

The complex interrelationships between different atopic manifestations at different ages and immune dysfunction, including atopic sensitization, are by no means clear. In most prevention studies, probiotics have not reduced atopic sensitization assessed by either skin prick testing or serum levels of allergen-specific IgE antibodies, this even despite positive effects on eczema incidence (see **Table 1**). Furthermore, in the study with thus far the longest reported follow-up to the age of 7 years probiotics were not shown to protect from food allergy or reduce asthma risk.[43–45] Fundamental questions regarding the nature and pathogenesis of atopic disease thus remain to be solved before a comprehensive understanding of probiotic effects may be reached. The same holds true for the interpretation of the effects of probiotics in the treatment of these disorders.

Impact of Probiotics in Established Allergic Disease

There are several reports of clinical trials in which probiotics have been used to alleviate symptoms of atopic eczema or food allergy. Notwithstanding recent meta-analyses with the inherent problems discussed previously,[59,60] extensively hydrolyzed formula supplemented with either *L rhamnosus* GG or *Bifidobacterium lactis* Bb-12 has been reported to be associated with a significant alleviation of atopic eczema symptoms accompanied by a reduction in intestinal and systemic allergic inflammation compared with infants receiving unsupplemented formula.[61–63] Similar results have been obtained using different *Lactobacillus* strains in older children with atopic eczema, with a most pronounced effect in children with detectable IgE sensitization.[64] In line with this observation, *L rhamnosus* GG reportedly alleviates eczema symptoms in IgE-sensitized infants but not in those without sensitization[65]; and the combination of *L rhamnosus* and *B lactis* has been detected to improve eczema in food sensitized but not in nonsensitized children.[66] Because *L rhamnosus* GG has been observed to improve the skin condition of infants with cow's milk allergy and atopic eczema[61,62]

Table 1
Double-blind, placebo-controlled clinical trials assessing efficacy of probiotics in reducing the risk of eczema in infants.

Study	N	Disease Risk	Probiotics	Intervention	Follow-up	Sensitization	Eczema
Kalliomäki et al[43–45]	159	Family history	LGG[a] of atopic disease	Mother 2–4 wk before delivery Mother/child 6 mo	7 y mother/child	No effect 6 mo	Significantly reduced by probiotics
Taylor et al[46]	231	Sensitized mothers with allergic disease	L acidophilus[b]	Child 6 mo	12 mo	Significantly increased by probiotics	No effect
Kukkonen et al[47]	1223	Parent with atopic disease	LGG[a] L rhamnosus[c] B breve[d] Pr freudenreichii[e] prebiotics	Mother 2–4 wk before delivery Child 6 mo	5 y	No effect	Significantly reduced by probiotics at 2 y, no effect at 5 y
Abrahamsson et al[48]	232	Family history of atopic disease	L reuteri[f]	Mother 4 wk before delivery Child 12 mo	12 mo	No effect	No effect on eczema, IgE-mediated eczema reduced by probiotics
Wickens et al[49]	474	Parent with atopic disease	L rhamnosus[g] or B animalis[h]	Mother 5 wk before delivery Mother during breastfeeding Child 2 y	2 y	No effect	Significantly reduced
Kopp et al[50]	105	Family history of atopic disease	LGG[a]	Mother 4–6 wk before delivery Mother/child 6 mo	2 y	No effect	No effect
Soh et al[51]	253	Family history of allergic disease	B longum[i] L rhamnosus[j]	Child 6 mo	12 mo	No effect	No effect
Niers et al[52]	156	Family history of atopic disease	B bifidum[k] B lactis[l] Lc lactis[m]	Mother 6 wk before delivery Child 12 mo	12 mo	No effect	Reduced at 3 mo No effect at 12 mo

Study	N	Population	Probiotic	Timing	Duration		
West et al[53]	179	Caesarian section delivery	LF19[n]	Child 4–13 mo	13 mo	No effect	Significantly reduced by probiotics
Dotterud et al[54]	415	Nonselected population	LGG[a] L acidophilus[o] B animalis[p]	Mother 4 wk before delivery Mother 3 mo while breastfeeding	2 y	No effect	Significantly reduced by probiotics
Kim et al[55]	112	Family history of allergic disease	B bifidum[q] B lactis[r] L acidophilus[s]	Mother 4–8 wk before delivery Mother 0–3 mo Child 4–6 mo	12 mo	No effect	Significantly reduced by probiotics
Boyle et al[56]	250	Family history of atopic disease	LGG[a]	Mother 4 wk before delivery	12 mo	No effect	No effect

[a] Lactobacillus rhamnosus GG (American Type Culture Collection 53103).
[b] Lactobacillus acidophilus (LAVRI-A1).
[c] L rhamnosus LC705 (DSM 7061).
[d] Bifidobacterium breve Bb99 (DSM 13,692).
[e] Propionibacterium freudenreichii ssp shermanii JS (DSM 7076).
[f] Lactobacillus reuteri (American Type Culture Collection 55730).
[g] L rhamnosus HN001.
[h] Bifidobacterium animalis subsp. lactis strain HN019.
[i] Bifidobacterium longum (BL999).
[j] L rhamnosus (LPR).
[k] Bifidobacterium bifidum W23.
[l] Bifidobacterium lactis W52.
[m] Lactococcus lactis W58.
[n] Lactobacillus F19.
[o] B animalis subsp. lactis Bb-12.
[p] L acidophilus La-5.
[q] B bifidum BGN4.
[r] B lactis AD011.
[s] L acidophilus AD031.

but to have no beneficial effect in infants with moderate eczema without gut involvement,[67,68] it may be suggested that probiotic effects on established eczema may be most pronounced in individuals with intestinal involvement or IgE sensitization. Future research should strive to objectively define target populations based on the precise clinical conditions, taking into account the clinical manifestations and immunologic mechanisms of the disease. Improved classification and understanding of the basic pathogenetic mechanism of atopic disorders are clearly called for.

FUTURE CHALLENGES

In the intestine's mucosa a balance is generated and maintained between the host and the microbiota. Moreover, the establishment of the gut microbiota provides an initial and massive source of microbial stimuli for the healthy maturation of the gut-associated lymphoid tissue. In fact, immune regulation in this interface unites the internal and external environments of the child. The intimate and multiple interrelationships between diet, the immune system, and the microbiome determines whether or not disease susceptibility manifests itself in chronic inflammatory disease later in life. To reverse such a progression, the joint action of specific nutrients and probiotics on the intestinal milieu can be therapeutically exploited, the rationale being restoration of the properties of the unbalanced indigenous microbiota, control of the inflammatory response, and tolerance induction. Before such measures can be put into practice, a better characterization of allergic conditions is essential, because there are distinct etiologic age-related factors and pathogenetic mechanisms underlying the heterogeneous manifestations of allergic disorders.

Taken together, several major challenges need to be met. Rigorous scientific efforts are needed to characterize the following:

- The sensitive stages of maturation
- How immunology is regulated during pregnancy and early infancy
- The immune interaction between nutritional and microbial factors
- How the regulation is related to disease risk
- The link between allergic conditions and other common chronic diseases rising in incidence world-wide
- The gut microbiota of the healthy breastfed child who also remains healthy long-term
- The microbiota in potential target organs in allergic conditions
- The probiotic potential of specific strains with anti-inflammatory and tolerogenic effects
- The mechanisms of the different allergic conditions, to provide specific targets for the most potent probiotics

SUMMARY

Recent demonstration that a growing number of clinical conditions, phenotypes as different as inflammatory bowel disease, obesity, and allergic diseases, are linked to aberrant gut microbiota composition has led to a resurgence of interest in host-microbe crosstalk, characterizing and manipulating the gut microbiota at an early age. The rationale of the approach is to avert immunoinflammatory responses, this subsequent to the recognition of the intimate interrelationship between diet, immune system, and microbiome and the origins of human disease. Abundant evidence implies that specific strains selected from the members of healthy gut microbiota exhibit powerful antipathogenic and anti-inflammatory capabilities, which may directly shape the risk of allergic disease during a critical period of life when the scene is set for the consolidation of the immune responder type. Notwithstanding that several aspects of the mechanisms of allergic diseases of diverse phenotype remain obscure, targets for the probiotic approach have emerged in established allergic disease: degradation/structural modification of enteral antigens, normalization of the properties of aberrant indigenous microbiota and of gut barrier functions, regulation of the secretion of proinflammatory mediators, and promotion of the maturation of the immune system. Current research is harnessing novel techniques to characterize the healthy gut microbiota, the source of probiotics, and the risk population, to optimize the mode of introducing the most efficient probiotic strains to those best profiting from them.

REFERENCES

1. Rautava S, Ruuskanen O, Ouwehand A, et al. The hygiene hypothesis of atopic disease: an extended version. J Pediatr Gastroenterol Nutr 2004;38:378–88.
2. Turnbaugh PJ, Ridaura VK, Faith JJ, et al. The effect of diet on the human gut microbiome: a metagenomic analysis in humanized gnotobiotic mice. Sci Transl Med 2009;1:6ra14.
3. Gerrard JW, Geddes CA, Reggin PL, et al. Serum IgE levels in white and metis communities in Saskatchewan. Ann Allergy 1976;37:91–100.
4. Strachan DP. Hay fever, hygiene, and household size. BMJ 1989;299:1259–60.
5. Hersoug LG, Linneberg A. The link between the epidemics of obesity and allergic diseases: does obesity induce decreased immune tolerance? Allergy 2007;62:1205–13.
6. Mai XM, Becker AB, Sellers EA, et al. The relationship of breast-feeding, overweight and asthma in preadolescents. J Allergy Clin Immunol 2007;120:551–6.
7. Kero J, Gissler M, Hemminki E, et al. Could the TH1 and TH2 diseases coexist? evaluation of asthma incidence in children with coeliac disease, type 1 diabetes or rheumatoid arthritis. A register study. J Allergy Clin Immunol 2001;108:781–3.
8. Kalliomäki M, Kirjavainen P, Eerola E, et al. Distinct patterns of neonatal gut microflora in infants in whom atopy was and was not developing. J Allergy Clin Immunol 2001;107:129–34.
9. Björkstén B, Sepp E, Julge K, et al. Allergy development and the intestinal microflora during the first year of life. J Allergy Clin Immunol 2001;108:516–20.
10. He F, Morita H, Hashimoto H, et al. Intestinal *Bifidobacterium* species induce varying cytokine production. J Allergy Clin Immunol 2002;109:1035–6.
11. Harris JK, Wagner BD. Bacterial identification and analytic challenges in clinical microbiome studies. J Allergy Clin Immunol 2012;129:441–2.
12. Renz H, von Mutius E, Brandtzaeg P, et al. Gene-environment interactions in chronic inflammatory disease. Nat Immunol 2011;12:273–7.
13. Clarke TB, Davis KM, Lysenko ES, et al. Recognition of peptidoglycan from the microbiota by Nod1 enhances systemic innate immunity. Nature Med 2010;16:228–31.
14. Maslowski KM, Vieira AT, Mg A, et al. Regulation of inflammatory responses by gut microbiota and chemoattractant receptor GPR43. Nature 2009;461:1282–6.
15. Cummings JH, Antoine JM, Aspiroz F, et al. PASSCLAIM (Process for the Assessment of Scientific Support for Claims on Foods): Gut health and immunity. Eur J Nutr 2004;43(Suppl 2):118–73.
16. Gallagher AM, Meijer GW, Richardson DP, et al. International Life Sciences Institute Europe Functional Foods Task Force. A standardised approach towards

PROving the efficacy of foods and food constituents for health CLAIMs (PROCLAIM): providing guidance. Br J Nutr 2011;106(Suppl 2):S16–28.

17. Welch RW, Antoine JM, Berta JL, et al. International Life Sciences Institute Europe Functional Foods Task Force. Guidelines for the design, conduct and reporting of human intervention studies to evaluate the health benefits of foods. Br J Nutr 2011;106(Suppl 2):S3–15.

18. Isolauri E, Kirjavainen PV, Salminen S. Probiotics: a role in the treatment of intestinal infection and inflammation? Gut 2002;50(Suppl III):54–9.

19. Favier CF, de Vos WM, Akkermans AD. Development of bacterial and bifidobacterial communities in feces of newborn babies. Anaerobe 2003;9:219–29.

20. Favier CF, Vaughan EE, De Vos WM, et al. Molecular monitoring of succession of bacterial communities in human neonates. Appl Environ Microbiol 2002;68: 219–26.

21. Palmer C, Bik EM, DiGiulio DB, et al. Development of the human infant intestinal microbiota. PLoS Biol 2007;5:e177. http://dx.doi.org/10.1371/journal.pbio.0050177.

22. Koenig JE, Spor A, Scalfone N, et al. Succession of microbial consortia in the developing infant gut microbiome. Proc Natl Acad Sci U S A 2011;108(Suppl 1):4578–85.

23. Mändar R, Livukene K, Ehrenberg A, et al. Amniotic fluid microflora in asymptomatic women at mid-gestation. Scand J Infect Dis 2001;33:60–2.

24. DiGiulio D. Diversity of microbes in amniotic fluid. Semin Fetal Neonatal Med 2012;17:2–11.

25. Onderdonk AB, Delaney ML, DuBois AM, et al. Detection of bacteria in placental tissues obtained from extremely low gestational age neonates. Am J Obstet Gynecol 2008;198:1–7.

26. Mshvildadze M, Neu J. The infant intestinal microbiome: friend or foe? Early Hum Dev 2010;86(Suppl 1):67–71.

27. Gueimonde M, Laitinen K, Salminen S, et al. Breast milk: a source of bifidobacteria for infant gut development and maturation? Neonatology 2007;92:64–6.

28. Perez PF, Doré J, Leclerc M, et al. Bacterial imprinting of the neonatal immune system: lessons from maternal cells? Pediatrics 2007;119:e724–32.

29. Cabrera-Rubio R, Collado MC, Laitinen K, et al. The human milk microbiome changes over lactation and is shaped by maternal weight and mode of delivery. Am J Clin Nutr 2012;96:544–51.

30. Grönlund MM, Gueimonde M, Laitinen K, et al. Maternal breast-milk and intestinal bifidobacteria guide the compositional development of the *Bifidobacterium* microbiota in infants at risk of allergic disease. Clin Exp Allergy 2007;37:1764–72.

31. Grönlund MM, Grzeskowiak L, Isolauri E, et al. Influence of mother's intestinal microbiota on gut colonisation in the infant. Gut Microbes 2011;2:227–33.

32. Collado MC, Isolauri E, Laitinen K, et al. Effect of mother's weight on infant's microbiota acquisition, composition, and activity during early infancy: a prospective follow-up study initiated in early pregnancy. Am J Clin Nutr 2010;92:1023–30.

33. Salminen S, Gibson GR, McCartney AL, et al. Influence of mode of delivery on gut microbiota composition in seven year old children. Gut 2004;53:1388–9.

34. Dominguez-Bello MG, Costello EK, Contreras M, et al. Delivery mode shapes the acquisition and structure of the initial microbiota across multiple body habitats in newborns. Proc Natl Acad Sci U S A 2010;107:11971–5.

35. Neu J, Rushing J. Cesarean versus vaginal delivery: long-term infant outcomes and the hygiene hypothesis. Clin Perinatol 2011;38:321–31.

36. van Nimwegen F, Penders J, Stobberingh E, et al. Mode and place of delivery, gastrointestinal microbiota, and their influence on asthma and atopy. J Allergy Clin Immunol 2011;128:948–55.e1–3.

37. WHO 2002. Guidelines for the evaluation of probiotics in food. Available at: http://www.who.int/foodsafety/publications/fs_management/probiotics2/en/. Accessed September 29, 2012.
38. Grześkowiak Ł, Isolauri E, Salminen S, et al. Manufacturing process influences properties of probiotic bacteria. Br J Nutr 2011;105:887–94.
39. Nivoliez A, Camares O, Paquet-Gachinat M, et al. Influence of manufacturing processes on in vitro properties of the probiotic strain *Lactobacillus rhamnosus* Lcr35. J Biotechnol 2012;160:236–41.
40. Tuomola E, Crittenden R, Playne M, et al. Quality assurance criteria for probiotic bacteria. Am J Clin Nutr 2001;73:393S–8S.
41. Isolauri E, Kalliomäki M, Laitinen K, et al. Modulation of the maturing gut barrier and microbiota: a novel target in allergic disease. Curr Pharm Des 2008;14:1368–75.
42. Deshpande G, Rao S, Patole S, et al. Updated meta-analysis of probiotics for preventing necrotizing enterocolitis in preterm neonates. Pediatrics 2010;125:921–30.
43. Kalliomäki M, Salminen S, Arvilommi H, et al. Probiotics in primary prevention of atopic disease: a randomised placebo-controlled trial. Lancet 2001;357:1076–9.
44. Kalliomäki M, Salminen S, Poussa T, et al. Probiotics and prevention of atopic disease: 4-year follow-up of a randomised placebo-controlled trial. Lancet 2003;361:1869–71.
45. Kalliomäki M, Salminen S, Poussa T, et al. Probiotics during the first 7 years of life: a cumulative risk reduction of eczema in a randomized, placebo-controlled trial. J Allergy Clin Immunol 2007;119:1019–21.
46. Taylor AL, Dunstan JA, Prescott SL. Probiotic supplementation for the first 6 months of life fails to reduce the risk of atopic dermatitis and increases the risk of allergen sensitization in high-risk children: a randomized controlled trial. J Allergy Clin Immunol 2007;119:184–91.
47. Kukkonen K, Savilahti E, Haahtela T, et al. Probiotics and prebiotic galacto-oligosaccharides in the prevention of allergic diseases: a randomized, double-blind, placebo-controlled trial. J Allergy Clin Immunol 2007;119:192–8.
48. Abrahamsson TR, Jakobsson T, Böttcher MF, et al. Probiotics in prevention of IgE-associated eczema: a double-blind, randomized, placebo-controlled trial. J Allergy Clin Immunol 2007;119:1174–80.
49. Wickens K, Black PN, Stanley TV, et al. A differential effect of 2 probiotics in the prevention of eczema and atopy: a double-blind, randomized, placebo-controlled trial. J Allergy Clin Immunol 2008;122:788–94.
50. Kopp MV, Hennemuth I, Heinzmann A, et al. Randomized, double-blind, placebo-controlled trial of probiotics for primary prevention: no clinical effects of *Lactobacillus* GG supplementation. Pediatrics 2008;121:e850–6.
51. Soh SE, Aw M, Gerez I, et al. Probiotic supplementation in the first 6 months of life in at risk Asian infants: effects on eczema and atopic sensitization at the age of 1 year. Clin Exp Allergy 2009;39:571–8.
52. Niers L, Martín R, Rijkers G, et al. The effects of selected probiotic strains on the development of eczema (the PANDA study). Allergy 2009;64:1349–58.
53. West CE, Hammarström ML, Hernell O. Probiotics during weaning reduce the incidence of eczema. Pediatr Allergy Immunol 2009;20:430–7.
54. Dotterud CK, Storrø O, Johnsen R, et al. Probiotics in pregnant women to prevent allergic disease: a randomized, double-blind trial. Br J Dermatol 2010;163:616–23.
55. Kim JY, Kwon JH, Ahn SH, et al. Effect of probiotic mix (*Bifidobacterium bifidum*, *Bifidobacterium lactis*, *Lactobacillus acidophilus*) in the primary prevention of

eczema: a double-blind, randomized, placebo-controlled trial. Pediatr Allergy Immunol 2010;21:e386–93.

56. Boyle RJ, Ismail IH, Kivivuori S, et al. *Lactobacillus* GG treatment during pregnancy for the prevention of eczema: a randomized controlled trial. Allergy 2011;66:509–16.

57. Doege K, Grajecki D, Zyriax BC, et al. Impact of maternal supplementation with probiotics during pregnancy on atopic eczema in childhood: a meta-analysis. Br J Nutr 2012;107:1–6.

58. Rautava S, Kalliomäki M, Isolauri E. Probiotics during pregnancy and breast-feeding might confer immunomodulatory protection against atopic disease in the infant. J Allergy Clin Immunol 2002;109:119–21.

59. Boyle RJ, Bath-Hextall FJ, Leonardi-Bee J, et al. Probiotics for treating eczema. Cochrane Database Syst Rev 2008;4:CD006135.

60. Boyle RJ, Bath-Hextall FJ, Leonardi-Bee J, et al. Probiotics for the treatment of eczema: a systematic review. Clin Exp Allergy 2009;39:1117–27.

61. Majamaa H, Isolauri E. Probiotics: a novel approach in the management of food allergy. J Allergy Clin Immunol 1997;99:179–85.

62. Isolauri E, Arvola T, Sütas Y, et al. Probiotics in the management of atopic eczema. Clin Exp Allergy 2000;30:1604–10.

63. Pessi T, Sütas Y, Hurme M, et al. Interleukin-10 generation in atopic children following oral *Lactobacillus rhamnosus* GG. Clin Exp Allergy 2000;30:1804–8.

64. Rosenfeldt V, Benfeldt E, Nielsen SD, et al. Effect of probiotic *Lactobacillus* strains in children with atopic dermatitis. J Allergy Clin Immunol 2003;111: 389–95.

65. Viljanen M, Savilahti E, Haahtela T, et al. Probiotics in the treatment of atopic eczema/dermatitis syndrome in infants: a double-blind placebo-controlled trial. Allergy 2005;60:494–500.

66. Sistek D, Kelly R, Wickens K, et al. Is the effect of probiotics on atopic dermatitis confined to food sensitized children? Clin Exp Allergy 2006;36:629–33.

67. Gruber C, Wendt M, Sulser C, et al. Randomized, placebo-controlled trial of *Lactobacillus* GG as treatment of atopic dermatitis in infancy. Allergy 2007;62: 1270–6.

68. Brouwer ML, Wolt-Plompen SA, Dubois AE, et al. No effects of probiotics on atopic dermatitis in infancy: a randomized placebo-controlled trial. Clin Exp Allergy 2006;36:899–906.

The Role of Probiotics in the Prevention and Treatment of Antibiotic-Associated Diarrhea and Clostridium Difficile Colitis

Gerald Friedman, MD, PhD, MS, MACG, AGAF

KEYWORDS

- Probiotics • Diarrhea • Antibiotic • Leukocytosis

KEY POINTS

- The spectrum of antibiotic-associated diarrhea (AAD) ranges from self-limited diarrheal episodes without complications to antibiotic-associated colitis.
- Ten percent to twenty five percent of all cases of AAD are due to overgrowth of C. difficile.
- Disruption of the protective colonic flora by broad spectrum antibiotics is the commonest predisposing factor to Clostridium difficile infection (CDI).
- The rate and severity of C. difficile has increased nationally and worldwide in part related to a new hyper virulent strain NAPI/BI/027.
- The 3 central features predisposing to CDI are immune-suppressed, elderly, hospitalized patients exposed to antibiotics.
- Meta-analyses and randomized controlled trials (RCTs) confirm the value of probiotics, particularly Saccharomyces boulardii and Lactobacillus GG, in the prevention of AAD.
- A single, dose-ranging RCT, using a probiotic mixture of L. acidophilus CL1285 and L.casei LBC80R, significantly prevented CDI.

INTRODUCTION

Diarrhea is one of the most frequent side effects of antibiotic use. The incidence of antibiotic-associated diarrhea (AAD) varies between 5% and 39% of patients, with a higher percentage seen in hospitalized patients.[1]

AAD is defined as otherwise unexplained diarrhea that occurs in association with the administration of antibiotics. It is characterized by a change in the normal stool frequency with at least 3 loose or watery stools daily for 3 days. Early onset of diarrhea

Department of Medicine, The Mount Sinai School of Medicine, 1 Gustave L. Levy Place, New York City, NY 10029, USA
E-mail address: gfmd379@gmail.com

Gastroenterol Clin N Am 41 (2012) 763–779
http://dx.doi.org/10.1016/j.gtc.2012.08.002
0889-8553/12/$ – see front matter © 2012 Elsevier Inc. All rights reserved.

occurs within 2 to 7 days, being earlier with children than outpatient adults. Delayed onset of diarrhea may occur within 2 to 8 weeks after the antibiotic has been discontinued.

Special attention should be accorded to at-risk hospitalized patients who may develop Clostridium difficile infection (CDI) complicating AAD. Prompt stool analysis for toxins A and B is essential for these patients. At-risk patients for CDI include patients aged greater than 65 years, patients with multiple comorbidities, immunosuppression, exposure to radiation and chemotherapy, inflammatory bowel disease (IBD), hepatic cirrhosis, prolonged hospitalization, and treatment with proton pump inhibitors (PPIs) (**Box 1**). Pharmacologically, the use of broad spectrum antibiotics and the duration of antibiotic therapy increase risk of AAD.

CAUSES OF AAD

Antibiotics cause diarrhea by several mechanisms.[2] First, suppression of anaerobic bacteria results in reduced metabolism of carbohydrates inducing an osmotic diarrhea. Secondly, antibiotics disrupt the protective effect of commensal bacteria. The disruption of microbial diversity reduces colonic mucosal resistance to pathogenic opportunistic bacteria, particularly CDI.[3] Following discontinuation of the antibiotic, restoration of the normal commensal bacteria may take several weeks, months, or longer to occur, thus placing the patient at longer term risk for disease-causing pathogenic agents. Finally, antibiotics with prokinetic activity, such as erythromycin and clavulanate, promote diarrhea.

PREVENTING AAD WITH PROBIOTICS

Multiple studies support the use of probiotics for preventing AAD. AAD presents a fertile area to study the efficacy of probiotics.[4] The study design is simplified because diarrhea is a predictable side effect; the impact of the antibiotic usually occurs early in the course of administration; the duration of therapy is usually limited (eg, 10–14 days), and, in most instances, the side effects of added probiotics are

---

Box 1
Risk factors for CDI

Hospitalization

Age greater than 65 years

Multiple comorbidities

Immunosuppression

Exposure to radiation

Chemotherapy

Prolonged hospitalization

Inflammatory bowel disease

Hepatic cirrhosis

Antibiotic therapy

Proton pump inhibitors

Prior history of CDI

Use of fluoroquinolones

minimal. In addition, given the spectrum of AAD, possibly eventuating to the more serious CDI, an effective probiotic represents a major step in reducing more serious illness. Most studies, both in children and adults, have been reported with positive results. Interpretation of studies is difficult partly because of the varied populations, age of the patients, comorbidities, drug interactions, duration of probiotic administration, numbers of patients involved, the nature and dose of the offending antibiotic agent, and the lack of randomized, placebo-controlled trials (**Box 2**). Clinically acceptable probiotics must be species specific; of human origin; survive passage from the oral cavity through the gastric acid barrier, digestive enzymes, and bile acids; travel down the small bowel into the colon; nidate; and proliferate therein. Probiotics should be of adequate dose, preferably greater than 10 billion cfu/gm in adults, maintain their viability and concentration, and have a dependably measurable shelf life at the time of purchase and administration (**Box 3**). When these qualities have been met, targeted illnesses require randomized, placebo-controlled, double-blinded trials on appropriate populations.

MECHANISMS OF ACTION OF PROBIOTICS

Probiotics offer protection from potential pathogens by enhancing mucosal barrier function by secreting mucins, providing colonization resistance, producing bacteriocins, increasing production of secretory immunoglobulin A (IgA), producing a balanced T-helper cell response, and increasing production of interleukin 10 (IL-10) and transforming growth factor beta, both of which play a role in the development of immunologic tolerance to antigens (**Box 4**).[5]

SINGLE STRAIN PROBIOTICS USED FOR TREATING AAD
Lactobacillus GG

Gorbach[6] began a search for the "ideal" lactobacillus by listing the biologic characteristics of a probiotic that would benefit human health. He collected strains of lactobacilli from stool specimens of healthy human volunteers. Each strain needed to survive the impact of gastric acid, bile acids, and pancreatic proteolytic enzymes; transit the small bowel to the colon where it would adhere to intestinal cells; colonize; and proliferate. The strain has to be safe, have good growth characteristics, and produce an antibacterial substance. The strain having the fastest growth and possessing the other characteristics was identified in 1985 and was named Lactobacillus GG (LGG) after its discoverers. LGG produces an inhibitory substance with activity against a variety of bacterial species, including anaerobic bacteria. LGG can be cultured in stool for 7 days after administration and from intestinal biopsy specimens for 28 days.

Box 2
Problems assessing probiotic publications
Insufficient number of trial patients
Variable ages of patients
Multiple comorbidities
Varied nature and dose of offending antibiotic
Different durations of probiotic administration
Lack of randomized, placebo-controlled trials

> **Box 3**
> **Characteristics of clinically acceptable probiotics**
>
> Species specific
>
> Human Origin
>
> Survive passage gastric, small bowel to colon, nidate/proliferate
>
> Adequate dosage; preferably greater than 10 billion CFU/g
>
> Maintain viability and concentration from time of purchase
>
> Dependably measurable shelf life
>
> Requires randomized, double-blind, placebo-controlled trials

Saccharomyces Boulardii

Saccharomyces boulardii, a probiotic yeast, was discovered in 1920 by the microbiologist Henri Boulard when he was in Indochina. He noted that during an epidemic of cholera, the natives who ingested a special tea did not develop this diarrheal illness. The tea was made by cooking the outer skin of lychee and mangosteens. Boulard succeeded in isolating the responsible agent, a special strain of yeast, which he named *Saccharomyces* boulardii.

In 1947, the patent for the yeast was purchased by Laboratories Biocodex, which initiated research and manufacturing protocols.[7] The lyophilized product, in capsule form, is stable at room temperature for more than 1 year. This preparation survives the actions of acid, bile acids, and proteolytic enzymes in its passage to the colon. Steady state concentrations are achieved in a mean of 3 days, and the cells are cleared from the stools from 2 to 5 days after discontinuation.

The mechanisms of action of S. boulardii include antitoxin effects by blocking pathogen toxin receptor sites or direct destruction of the toxin as exemplified by the degradation of toxins A and B of C. difficile and by reducing the effect of cholera toxin. S. boulardii interferes with the growth of several pathogens including Candida albicans, Salmonella typhimurium, Yersinia enterocolitica, and Alpha hemolysin. The yeast may also protect the integrity of epithelial tight junctions, reducing permeability to potential pathogens. In addition, S. boulardii has been demonstrated to increase the recovery rate of bacterial flora following the impact of antibiotics on the commensal flora.

S. boulardii is resistant to antibacterial agents. The yeast may cause an increase in secretory IgA levels and may act as an immune stimulant by reducing proinflammatory responses.

> **Box 4**
> **Mechanisms of action of probiotics**
>
> Enhancing mucosal barrier function by secreting mucins
>
> Increasing tight junctions
>
> Providing colonization resistance
>
> Producing bacteriocins
>
> Increasing production of secretory IgA
>
> Producing a balanced T-helper cell response
>
> Increase production of IL-10 and transforming growth factor beta

MULTISTRAIN PROBIOTICS FOR TREATING AAD
L. Casei, S. Thermophilus, and L. Bulgaricus

S. thermophilus and L. bulgaricus are used to produce yogurt by the fermentation of lactic acid.[8] More recently, 2 combined lactobacillus strains, L. casei and L. acidophilus, have been shown to be effective in a dose response manner to dramatically reduce AAD.[9] A smaller study of this agent was also used during a 2003 to 2004 endemic of CDI in Quebec Canada with beneficial results.[10]

PREVENTION OF PEDIATRIC AAD

Six placebo-controlled, RCTs comprising 766 children were included in a meta-analysis of probiotics preventing AAD that was published in 2006.[11] Treatment with probiotics compared with placebo reduced the risk of AAD from 28.5% to 11.9%. Pre-planned subgroup analysis showed that reduction of the risk of AAD was associated with the use of LGG, S. boulardii, or B. lactis, and Streptococcus thermophilus. Probiotics reduced the risk of AAD in children; of every 7 patients who would develop diarrhea while being treated with antibiotics, one fewer will develop AAD if also receiving probiotics.

No adverse effects were observed in any of the included trials. However, the investigators cautioned regarding the use of probiotics in immune-compromised patients. They recommended identification of populations at high risk of AAD who would benefit most from use of probiotic therapy, assessment of additional probiotic strains, designing an effective dosing regimen, and addressing the cost effectiveness of using probiotics to prevent AAD in children.

A Cochrane Database review of the data on probiotics in preventing pediatric AAD was published in 2011.[12] Sixteen studies were reviewed and provided the best available evidence. The studies tested 3432 children (2 weeks to 17 years of age) who were receiving probiotics coadministered with antibiotics to prevent AAD. These short-term studies showed probiotics to be effective for preventing AAD. Probiotics were generally well tolerated (no significant side effects between probiotics and control groups). Both L. rhamnosus and S. boulardii at dosages of 5 to 40 billion CFU/d may prevent the onset of ADD, with no serious side effects in otherwise healthy children. This benefit for high-dose probiotics needs to be confirmed by a large randomized study. No conclusions regarding other probiotic agents could be drawn.

PREVENTING ADULT AAD

Compiling data referable to the efficacy of probiotics suppressing AAD in adults is complicated by numerous factors. Variations in the clinical setting (hospitalized or community), numbers and ages of patients, nature of the population, type of antibiotic, duration of therapy, use of different probiotics, failure to designate the strain, variable dosages, and duration of therapy are some of the major factors making statistical judgment difficult. Three meta-analyses have been published in an effort to obtain useful clinical data. In 2002, D'Souza and colleagues[13] and Cremonini and colleagues[14] combined 9 and 7 trials, respectively.

In the D'Souza study, 2 of the 9 studies investigated the effects of probiotics in children. Four trials used S. boulardii, 4 used lactobacilli, and one used a strain of enterococcus that produced lactic acid. Three trials used a combination of probiotic strains of bacteria. The probiotics were given in combination with antibiotics, whereas the control groups received placebo and antibiotics. The odds ratio (OR) in favor of active treatment over placebo was 0.39 (95% confidence interval [CI], 0.25–0.62, $P<.001$) for the yeast and 0.34 (0.19–0.61, $P<.01$) for lactobacilli. The combined OR was 0.37 (0.26–0.53; $P<.001$) in favor of active treatment over placebo.

The investigators concluded that biotherapeutic agents may be useful in preventing AAD. Cremonini and colleagues (vide supra) limited their meta-analysis to 7 trials, which used the 2 most widely used probiotics Lactobacillus spp. and S. boulardii. Two studies involved children; 3 assessed the decrease in the occurrence of AAD during the administration of S. boulardii, and 4 during the administration of Lactobacillus spp. The search was limited to randomized studies. The inclusion criteria included a placebo design, with diarrhea as a primary end-point and a minimum of 2 weeks of follow-up. A total number of 881 patients were studied. The combined relative risk (RR) was 0.3966 (95% CI, 0.27–0.57). The results suggested a strong benefit of probiotic administration on AAD.

META-ANALYTIC POOLING

A large and comprehensive meta-analysis pooling trials of probiotics in the prevention of pediatric and adult AAD was accomplished by McFarland[15] in 2006. Study selection included trials in which specific probiotics were given to either prevent or treat the diseases of interest.

Trials were required to be randomized, blinded, controlled in humans, and published in peer-reviewed journals. Thirty one of 180 screened studies, totaling 3164 subjects, met the inclusion and exclusion criteria. From 25 RCTs (2810 patients), probiotics significantly reduced the RR of AAD (RR = 0.43, 95% CI, 0.31–0.58, $P<.001$).

Six of the trials, which included 1119 patients, used S. boulardii as the probiotic. One of the trials involved the use of triple antibiotics with concomitant S. boulardii for the eradication of Helicobacter pylori (43 patients). The same probiotic was used in a 246 pediatric patient trial. Six trials used LGG as the single probiotic; 388 pediatric patients in 3 trials, 267 adult patients in one trial, and 262 patients involved in 3 triple antibiotic/LLG trials for the eradication of H. pylori.

Overall, of 16 RCTs of adult AAD, 7 (44%) showed efficacy, whereas 9 RCTs (67%) showed significant efficacy in children. Of note, optimal results occurred with dosages of probiotics greater than 10^{10} cfu/g. Sixteen of 31 (84%) trials reported on adverse effects. In 24 trials, there were no adverse episodes. Nine percent of patients on S. boulardii reported increased thirst and 14% reported increased constipation. Thirty seven percent of patients on LGG reported mild gaseousness and 25% noted bloating.

AAD AND HELICOBACTER PYLORI THERAPY

A recent review of S. boulardii[16] included 3 trials conducted in patients with H. pylori infection. These patients were treated with triple therapy, which includes 2 antibiotics and a PPI for 2 weeks.

Duman and colleagues[17] treated 204 patients with 1 g of S. boulardii (2×10^{10}/d for 2 weeks) and triple therapy compared with 185 patients who received only triple therapy. Of the 389 patients, 376 completed the treatment phase and the 4-week follow-up. Fewer patients given S. boulardii (6.9%) developed AAD compared with the control group (15.6%, $P = .007$).

Two other RCTs were conducted in adult patients receiving triple therapy for H. pylori infections and both showed a significant reduction in AAD for those treated with S. boulardii.[18,19] In summary, the use of concomitant probiotic therapy in association with multiple antibiotics and PPIs is helpful in reducing the antibiotic-induced gastrointestinal side effects.

META-ANALYTIC CONFIRMATION OF RESULTS SUPPORTING USE OF PROBIOTICS FOR AAD

A statistically sophisticated meta-analysis adding confirmation for the use of probiotics for treatment of AAD was published in April, 2012 by Videlock and Cremonini.[20] They used a meta-analysis of randomized, double-blinded, placebo-controlled trials including patients treated with antibiotics and administered a probiotic for at least the duration of the antibiotic treatment.

Meta-analysis and meta-regression methods were used to synthesize data and to assess influence of mean age, duration of antibiotics, risk of bias, and incidence of diarrhea in the placebo group on outcomes. Subgroup analyses explored effects of different probiotic species, patient populations, and treatment indications.

Thirty four studies were included with 4138 patients. Pooled RR for AAD in the probiotic group versus placebo was 0.53 (95% CI, 0.44–0.63), corresponding to a number needed to treat (NNT) of 8 (95% CI, 7–11). Pooled RR for AAD during treatment of H. pylori was 0.37 (95% CI, 0.20–0.69), with an NNT of 5 (95% CI, 4–10). This updated meta-analysis confirmed the results enumerated, supporting the effects of probiotics in AAD. Studies on the effect of probiotics in preventing the occurrence or reoccurrence of Clostridium difficile colitis were not included and will be discussed later in this article.

AAD–THE PATHWAY TO CLOSTRIDIUM DIFFICILE COLITIS

The spectrum of AAD ranges from self-limited diarrheal episodes without complications to antibiotic-associated colitis. Ten percent to 25% of all cases of AAD are due to overgrowth of C. difficile.[21]

C. difficile is an anaerobic, gram-positive spore-forming rod that colonizes the intestinal tract after alteration of the normal gastrointestinal flora. Disruption of the protective colonic flora by broad spectrum antibiotics is the commonest predisposing factor to CDI by altering "colonization resistance."

The extent of this disruption varies among individuals with restoration of normal flora usually taking 1 month after discontinuation of the antibiotic. However, in some instances it may take 6 months or longer.[22] It is now well established that antibiotic treatment increases susceptibility to enteric infections.[23]

C. difficile is the most common infectious disease affecting the gastrointestinal tract. It occurs in 8% to 10% of hospitalized patients and is responsible for 20% to 30% of cases of hospital-acquired diarrhea. The infection is mediated by 2 exotoxins, A and B, causing diarrhea and colonic mucosal inflammation. The spectrum of the disease varies from mild diarrhea to severe fulminant watery diarrhea associated with fever, leukocytosis, abdominal pain, distention, and hypoalbuminemia.

The rate and severity of C. difficile has increased nationally and worldwide in part related to a new hyper virulent strain, initially described in early 2000 in Quebec, Canada and the University of Pittsburgh Medical Center, USA.[24,25] Molecular analysis was characterized as group B1 by restriction endonuclease analysis, as North American pulse-field type NAP1, as pulse-field electrophoresis, and as ribotype 027.[26] The new strain is characterized by greater toxicity, a significant increase in toxins A and B, a higher rate of recurrent disease, and reduced response to metronidazole.

THE SPECTRUM OF CDI INFECTION

The spectrum of disease varies from an asymptomatic carrier state to mild diarrhea or life-threatening fulminant diarrhea and colitis. The carrier state affects approximately 20% of hospitalized patients. Although asymptomatic, they serve as a reservoir for environmental contamination. An even greater number of carrier patients are seen among nursing homes and long-term health facilities.[27]

Typical inhospital presentation is an elderly (>65 years of age) patient with an exposure to an antibiotic within the past 2 months presenting with frequent watery diarrhea for 2 to 3 days in association with crampy abdominal pain, nausea, and anorexia. Laboratories reveal leukocytosis, elevated C-reactive protein (CRP) level, and hypoalbuminemia. Stool examination result is positive for toxins A and B. The patient is placed in an isolation room and immediately treated with vancomycin 125 mg orally 4 times daily and carefully assessed on a daily basis.

Risk factors for inhospital patients include age greater than 65 years, male gender, immunodeficiency, multiple comorbidities, increased length of hospital stay, prolonged antibiotic use, antineoplastic medications, use of PPIs, use of fluoroquinolones, and the presence of IBD.

Community risk factors include pregnant and peripartum women, diminished immune status, nursing home patients, and IBD. A typical community patient would be a 26-year-old woman with a history of quiescent ulcerative colitis with no antibiotic exposure who experiences an acute flare with sudden onset of bloody diarrhea, fever, and leukocytosis. Stool analysis result is positive for toxins A and B. The patient is placed on metronidazole, 500 mg, 3 times daily, fluid, and electrolyte replacement and observed carefully for early signs of improvement; if no improvement occurs within 48 to 72 hours, the patient should receive 250 mg of vancomycin 4 times daily.

CLASSIFICATION OF DISEASE SEVERITY

Milder cases include low-grade diarrhea and less-systemic symptoms, including low-grade temperature, fewer cramps, and minimal leukocytosis. Colonic mucosal biopsies reveal inflammatory changes confined to the superficial epithelium and lamina propria with few crypt abscesses.

More advanced cases are exemplified by increased diarrheal episodes (>10–15 stools/d), greater abdominal pain, fever, and leukocytosis averaging 15,000. Mucosal biopsies are characterized by severe glandular disruption, crypt abscesses, and increased mucus secretion.

Fulminant colitis is characterized by severe lower abdominal pain and distention. Marked diarrhea is present followed by hypovolemia, lactic acidosis, hypoalbuminemia, and toxic mega colon, which may lead to perforation. Leukocytosis greater than 30,000 is a poor prognostic sign. Histopathology reveals intense necrosis involving full thickness of the mucosa with confluent pseudomembranes.

DIAGNOSIS OF CDI

Diagnosis should be suspected in any patient (especially elderly) developing clinically significant acute diarrhea within 2 months of antibiotic use or within 3 days of hospital admission. Clinically significant diarrhea is defined as 3 or more loose stools daily for at least 2 days. Additional important features of the patient's history include use of current medication, particularly immunosuppressives, PPIs, or steroid therapy.

A review of comorbidities is necessary with special attention to IBD and recent pregnancy. An allergic history and a prior history of C. difficile infection are important. A nutrition history, including weight loss and food and water intake, is essential. The differential diagnosis includes other enteric pathogens that can cause diarrhea, which includes salmonella, C. perfringens type A, Staphylococcus aureus, C. albicans, Campylobacter, and Shigella.

Travelers' diarrhea should be considered in patients with a recent history of foreign travel. Noninfectious diseases including irritable bowel syndrome, celiac disease, drug-induced diarrhea, and so on should be ruled out.

Major findings on physical examination include direct lower abdominal tenderness in association with fever and dehydration. Bedside sigmoidoscopic examination in an isolation room may reveal findings from mild patchy erythema and friability to marked edema, plaque formation, and severe pseudomembranous colitis. Stool guaiac test results are generally positive. Leukocytosis and hypoalbuminemia may be notable.

LABORATORY DIAGNOSIS

A complete blood count may reveal anemia (microcytic, hypochromic) and leukocytosis (elevated neutrophils) secondary to inflammation, hypovolemia (secondary to protein loss/diarrhea), and possible electrolyte imbalance. CRP level may be elevated. Stool examination may reveal stool leukocytes. Testing for toxins A and B (performed only on diarrheal stools) include enzyme immunoassay (EIA), which is rapid, but less sensitive than cell cytotoxin assay and polymerase chain reaction testing, which is rapid, sensitive, and specific.

Repeat testing during the same episode of diarrhea is usually of limited value. Imaging: plain films may be helpful to determine toxic mega colon or perforation. Abdominal computed tomography scan in patients with pseudomembranous colitis reveals thickening of the abdominal wall.

TREATMENT OF CDI

The primary goal for treatment of clostridium difficile colitis is to commence therapy, preferably as soon as the diagnosis is confirmed.[24,28]

- If diagnostic tests are unavailable, when severe or complicated CDI is suspected, empirical therapy should be initiated.
- If the result of stool toxin assay is negative, the decision to start therapy must be individualized. Discontinue therapy with the inciting antibiotic agent as soon as possible.
- Institute supportive care including hydration and electrolyte replacement. Avoid use of antiperistaltic medication (narcotics and anticholinergics).
- For mild to moderate initial episode of CDI, metronidazole is the drug of choice. The recommended dosage is 500 mg 3 times daily for 10 to 14 days.
- The exception is the presence of the virulent strain NAP1/BI/027, which may be resistant to metronidazole. Vancomycin orally in a dosage of 125 mg 4 times daily for 10 to 14 days should be substituted.
- Vancomycin is the drug of choice for initial episode of severe CDI. The dosage is 125 to 250 mg orally 4 times daily for 10 to 14 days. Vancomycin is given orally (and per rectum, if ileus is present), with or without intravenously administered metronidazole, is the regimen of choice for severe, complicated CDI.
- The vancomycin dosage is 500 mg orally 4 times daily and 500 mg in 100 mL normal saline rectally every 6 hours as a retention enema.
- The metronidazole dosage is 500 mg intravenously every 8 hours.
- Surgical consultation should be obtained early in the course of severe, complicated CDI.[29]
- Colectomy should be considered for severely ill patients. The patient's overall condition, an elevated serum lactate rising to 5 mmol/L and a white blood cell count (WBC) rising to 50 thousand cells/uL have been associated with increased

perioperative mortality. If surgical intervention is indicated, a subtotal colectomy with rectal preservation is recommended.

OTHER THERAPEUTIC CONSIDERATIONS

The search for new antimicrobial agents against C. difficile is driven by a desire to find an alternative to metronidazole and vancomycin, both as treatment of the acute inflammatory process, and to prevent recurrent episodes of colitis.

A recent Cochrane Review[30] investigated the efficacy of antibiotic therapy for C. difficile-associated diarrhea. Only RCTs assessing antibiotic treatment of CDI were included in the review. Fifteen studies with a total of 1152 participants with CDI were included. Nine different antibiotics were investigated: vancomycin, metronidazole, fusidic acid, nitazoxanide, teicoplanin, rifampin, rifaximin, bacitracin, and fidaxomicin. Most of these studies were active comparator studies comparing vancomycin with other antibiotics.

Vancomycin was found to be superior to placebo for improvement of symptoms of CDI including resolution of diarrhea. Most of the studies found no statistically significant difference in efficacy between vancomycin and other antibiotics. Many of these studies had small numbers of patients and suffered from methodological quality.

Teicoplanin, however, was found to be superior to vancomycin for curing the CDI. Teicoplanin is expensive and not readily available in the United States.[31]

The Food and Drug Administration has recently approved a new macrocyclic antibiotic with minimal systemic absorption, high fecal concentrations, and limited activity in vitro and in vivo against components of normal gut flora. The drug, fidaxomicin, has a narrow antimicrobial spectrum against gram-negative organisms and fungi. The dosage is 200 mg orally every 12 hours. The rates of cure with fidaxomicin were noninferior to vancomycin in the treatment of CDI. A multicenter trial with 629 patients also revealed a lower rate of recurrence of the infection.[32]

Tolevamer is a nonantibiotic, toxin-binding polymer, which noncovalently binds C. difficile toxins. This agent effectively treats mild to moderate C. difficile inflammation but does not alter commensal diversity.[33]

RECURRENT CLOSTRIDIUM DIFFICILE COLITIS

Recurrent C. difficile colitis occurs in 20% to 35% of patients with CDI, reflecting possible relapse of the original strain or reinfection with a new strain. Recurrence can occur within days to within 4 weeks following therapy with either metronidazole or vancomycin. The risk of recurrence is increased in patients who have already had one recurrence, rising from about 20% after an initial episode to about 40% after a first recurrence and to more than 60% after 2 or more recurrences.[34]

There are several suggested mechanisms explaining C. difficile relapses:

1. Reinfection may occur after initial clearance if there is repeat exposure in a contaminated environment because clostridial spores can persist in the environment allowing for exogenous reinfection.
2. Resistant spores may not have been destroyed during the initial antibiotic eradication of vegetative forms of C. difficile.[35]
3. The antibiotic triggering the acute infection may have dramatically altered the commensal bacteria to an extent that delayed homeostasis of the diverse protective bacteria, thus allowing the C. difficile vegetative form to proliferate.
4. Increased frequency of recurrences following metronidazole therapy.

5. Increased frequency of recurrences in patients older than 65 years of age.
6. Patients with a defective immune response to toxin A (**Box 5**).[36]

TREATMENT OF RECURRENT CDI

Vancomycin is recommended for the first recurrence in patients with a WBC of 15,000 cells/uL or higher or a rising serum creatinine level. A significant number of patients with a second recurrence will be cured with a tapering or pulsed regimen of oral vancomycin. After the initial dosage of 125 mg 4 times daily for 10 to 14 days, followed by 125 mg twice daily for 1 week, and then 125 mg every 3 days for 2 to 8 weeks.

Other potential options include other antimicrobial agents such as fidaxomicin, nitazoxanide, monoclonal antibody,[37] intravenous IgG,[38] the use of C. difficile toxoid vaccine,[39] or fecal transplantation.

Fecal biotherapy involves infusion of bacterial flora obtained from the feces of a healthy donor to reverse the bacterial imbalance responsible for the recurring nature of the infection. Donor stool is collected from a family member who has been tested for bacterial, viral, or parasitic pathogens. The stool is mixed with sterile saline and delivered through a nasogastric tube, colonoscopically or by retention enema. Published results of patients who have failed prior therapy report dramatic responses to this approach.[40]

INFECTION CONTROL AND PREVENTION MEASURES

The most important infection control and prevention measures include measures for patients, visitors, and health care workers; environmental cleaning; restrictions on antimicrobial agents; and the use of selected probiotics.

Infection spreads via the fecal-oral route. A patient-isolation room with a dedicated toilet is necessary; lid-down flushing is recommended. Hand washing with warm water and soap is indicated for patients, visitors, and health care providers.[41] The latter should be gloved and gowned appropriately.

Contact precautions should be maintained for the duration of diarrhea. Disposable medical equipment, including disposable rectal thermometers should be used. Chlorinated agents (with at least 1000 ppm available chlorine) should be used for effective room cleaning and disinfection. PPIs and antiperistaltic medications should be discontinued.

MONITORING ANTIMICROBIAL AGENTS

Antibiotic use is widely accepted as an important modifiable risk factor for C. difficile-associated diarrhea. The antibiotics most frequently implicated in the predisposition to

Box 5
Mechanisms contributing to recurrent CDI
Previous CDI infection
Repeat exposure to a contaminated environment
Resistant spores not destroyed during initial antibiotic eradication
Extreme and prolonged alteration of commensal bacterial flora with delayed restoration of flora
Age greater than 65 years
Patients with defective immune response to toxin A

CDI include fluoroquinolones, clindamycin, and broad spectrum penicillins and ceph-alosporins. Any antibiotic can disrupt the diversity of commensal bacteria and allow colonization by C. difficile.

The use of broad-spectrum antimicrobials, using multiple antibiotics, as well as pro-longed duration of antibiotic agents contribute to the increased incidence of CDI.[42] It is important to minimize the frequency and duration of antimicrobial agents in an effort to reduce the incidence of CDI. An antimicrobial stewardship program including phar-macy stop dates may be helpful.[43]

USING PROBIOTICS TO PREVENT CDI

The ideal probiotic preventing CDI is an agent that rapidly reduces AAD, prevents disruption of commensal bacteria, replaces previously depleted microflora, and returns microfloral functionality to the patient. The agent should be nontoxic, reason-ably priced, and readily available, with an acceptable shelf life and RCTs confirming its efficacy.

As noted previously, multiple clinical trials have confirmed the efficacy of various probiotics in the treatment of AAD. Thus, blocking the pathway from AAD to CDI reduces the ability of the vegetative form of the C. difficile organism break through the protective barrier of the intact protective commensal bacteria.

There are several recent randomized placebo-controlled studies that support this concept.[8] One thousand seven hundred and sixty patients were assessed for eligi-bility, of which 1625 were excluded. Total allocation included 135 patients, 69 in the probiotic group and 66 in the placebo group; including follow-up, the final analysis allowed for 57 patients in the probiotic group and 56 patients in the placebo group. The treatment group received a probiotic yogurt drink containing L. casei DN-114001 (L. casei Immunitas) $(1.0 \times 10^8$ cfu/mL), S. thermophilus $(1.0 \times 10^8$ cfu/mL), and L. bulgaricus $(1 \times 10^7$ cfu/mL). The placebo group received a long-life, sterile milkshake (Yazoo, Campina, Netherlands). Lactobacillus counts of the probiotic drinks were performed to ensure activity.

L. casei Immunitas had previously been shown to survive passage to the colon. Participants ingested the drinks within 48 hours of starting the antibiotic, continuing for 1 week after stopping the antibiotic. The participants drank 100 gm (97 mL) twice daily before or 1 to 2 hours after meals.

There were no reported adverse events related to the study drink. Most patients received an antibiotic, but about 40% received 2. The most common reasons for anti-biotic use were respiratory infections (49%) or prophylaxis before or after surgery (25%). Primary analysis was intention to treat.

There was a significant reduction in both the incidence of AAD $(P = .007)$ and C. difficile-associated diarrhea $(P = .001)$ in the probiotic group. The investigators concluded that consumption of a probiotic drink containing L. casei, L. bulgaricus, and S. thermophilus can reduce the incidence of AAD and C. difficile-associated diar-rhea, with the potential of decreasing morbidity, health care costs, and mortality if used routinely in patients aged more than 50 years. Three trials using another L. casei strain have been reported.

Two Canadian population studies were conducted with the primary objective of studying AAD and a secondary objective of determining the impact of the probiotic on CDI. The third study was a single center study performed on an Asian population (Shanghai).

A prospective, randomized, double-blind, placebo-controlled study was conducted at Maisonneuve-Rosemont Hospital, Montreal, Quebec.[10] Among 89 randomized, hospitalized patients, AAD occurred in 7 of 44 patients (15.9%) in the lactobacilli group and in 16 of 45 patients (35.6%) in the placebo group (OR 0.34, 95% CI, 0.125–0.944; $P = .05$). The median hospitalization duration was 8 days in the lactobacilli group compared with 10 days in the placebo group ($P = .09$). Lactobacilli fermented milk was well tolerated. Among all study patients, one patient in the lactobacilli group (2.3%) and 7 patients in the placebo group (15.6%) developed CDI (OR 0.126, 95% CI, 0.020–1.109; $P = .06$).

This study was followed by a Canadian centre study involving 216 patients randomized to L. acidophilus CL1285 and L. casei to placebo. The mean number of days with diarrhea was 1.19 (3.20) days for the placebo and 0.67 (2.05) days for the lactobacilli group ($P = .040$). Adjusted multivariate linear regression results showed that the duration of diarrhea for the lactobacillus group versus placebo was reduced by 51.5% (bSE) = 0.515 (0.0256), $P = .045$). The incidence of diarrhea was 21.8% for the lactobacilli group and 29.4% for the placebo group (OR = 0.667, $P = .067$). One patient in the Lactobacilli group was positive for C. difficile toxin as compared with 4 in the placebo group (OR = 0.433, $P = .645$).

Another randomized, double-blind, placebo-controlled, dose-ranging study added impetus to the Hickson study.[9] This single-center study randomized 255 adults in patients, aged 60 to 70 years, to 1 of 3 groups: 2 probiotic capsules consisting of 100 billion CFU/ml of the probiotic mixture L. acidophilus CL1285 and L. casei LBC8OR and one probiotic capsule containing 50 billion CFU/ml and one placebo capsule against group 3that includes 2 placebo capsules daily. Probiotic prophylaxis began within 36 hours of initial antibiotic administration and continued for 5 days after the last antibiotic dose. Patients took their daily dose 2 hours after breakfast and antibiotic administration each day. Patients were then observed for an additional 21 days.

Higher dose probiotic use had a lower AAD incidence compared with the lower dose probiotic (15.5% vs 28.2%, $P = .02$). Each probiotic group had a lower AAD incidence than placebo (44.1%, $P<.001$ for higher dose probiotic and $P = .02$ for lower dose probiotic). Patients on the probiotic had a shorter duration of symptoms. There was also a reduction in CDI incidence from 23.8% in the placebo group to 1.2% in the higher dose probiotic group ($P = .002$ vs placebo) and 9.4% in the lower dose probiotic group ($P = .03$ vs placebo). This report proved to be a classic dose-response result.

Despite the strain differences, L. casei was present in both studies. Further randomized studies would add to the value of both of these studies. The results of these studies compare favorably with a similar trial.[44] That study reported that patients taking a probiotic containing Lactobacillus and Bifidobacterium had a 2.9% CDI incidence versus 7.3% in a placebo group. The dose-response relationship implies that higher probiotic dosages may be associated with better outcomes. These studies also emphasize the value of prophylactic probiotic therapy in selected at-risk populations, particularly the elderly.

ADJUNCTIVE PROBIOTIC THERAPY TO PREVENT RECURRENT CDI

There is evidence suggesting that the yeast S. boulardii may reduce the incidence of recurrent CDI when adjunctively with high-dose vancomycin.[45]

SAFETY OF PROBIOTICS

The safety of probiotics is expertly reviewed in a separate article of this issue. Probiotics have an excellent overall safety record.[46] Major risk factors include immune compromise, premature infants. Minor risk factors include central venous catheter, altered epithelial barrier, jejunostomy feedings, and cardiac valvular disease or valvular replacement.

THE ECONOMIC IMPACT OF CLOSTRIDIUM DIFFICILE INFECTION

The incidence of CDI is increasing worldwide. This infectious illness has resulted in increased morbidity, mortality, and financial cost to the health care system. In fact, a large CDI economic evaluation confirmed that health care-associated cases of CDI are associated with significantly higher mean cost and longer length of stay than those of matched controls, with the greatest effect on costs at the lowest level of severity of illness.[47,48] This evaluation is further exacerbated by the increased recognition of the impact of CDI on patients, both children and adults with IBD.[49,50]

SUMMARY

Clearly, current evidence favors the use of probiotics in the prevention of symptoms of AAD. Lactobacilli, S. boulardii, and selected multistrain combinations, in appropriate dosages, are all clinically useful. The safety profile, with the exceptions noted earlier, is acceptable particularly in view of the short-term use of an antibiotic when accompanied by a probiotic. Recent statistical analysis substantiates this view.[51] Of greater importance is the compelling evidence that high-risk patients (especially the elderly) can prevent the morbidity and mortality related to CDI by using selected probiotics to block the pathway from AAD to CDI.

REFERENCES

1. McFarland LV. Antibiotic-associated diarrhea: epidemiology, trends and treatment. Future Microbiol 2008;3(5):563–78.
2. Doron SI, Hibberd PL, Gorbach SL. Probiotics for prevention of antibiotic-associated diarrhea. J Clin Gastroenterol 2008;42(Suppl 2):S58–63.
3. Young VB, Schmidt TM. Antibiotic-associated diarrhea accompanied by large-scale alterations in the composition of the fecal microbiota. J Clin Microbiol 2004;42(3):1203–6.
4. Surawicz CM. Role of probiotics in antibiotic-associated diarrhea, clostridium difficile associated diarrhea and recurrent clostridium difficile-associated diarrhea. J Clin Gastroenterol 2008;42(Suppl 2):S64–70.
5. Saavedra JM. Use of probiotics in pediatrics: rationale, mechanisms of action, and practical aspects. Nutr Clin Pract 2007;22:351–65.
6. Gorbach SL. The discovery of lactobacillus GG. Nutr Today 1996;31:25–45.
7. McFarland LV, Bernasconi P. Saccharomyces boulardii: a review of an innovative biotherapeutic agent. Microb Ecol Health Dis 1993;6:157–71.
8. Hickson M, D'Souza AL, Muthu N, et al. Use of probiotic lactobacillus preparation to prevent diarrhea associated with antibiotics: randomized double blind placebo controlled trial. BMJ 2007;335:80.
9. Gao XW, Mubasher M, Fang CY, et al. Dose-response efficacy of a proprietary probiotic formula of lactobacillus acidophilus CL1285 and lactobacillus casei LBC8oR for antibiotic-associated diarrhea and clostridium difficile-associated diarrhea prophylaxis in adult patients. Am J Gastroenterol 2010;105:1636–41.
10. Beausoleil M, Fortier N, Guenette S, et al. Effect of a fermented milk combining lactobacillus acidophilus CL1285 and lactobacillus casei in the prevention of antibiotic-associated diarrhea: a randomized, double-blind, placebo-controlled trial. Can J Gastroenterol 2007;21(11):732–6.

11. Szajewska H, Ruszczynski M, Radzkowski A. Probiotics in the prevention of antibiotic-associated diarrhea in children: a meta-analysis of randomized controlled trials. J Pediatr 2006;149:367–72.

12. Johnston BC, Goldenberg JZ, Vandvik PO, et al. Probiotics for the prevention of pediatric antibiotic-associated diarrhea. Cochrane Database Syst Rev 2011;(11):CD004827. http://dx.doi.org/10.1002/14651858.CD004827p.pub3.

13. D'Souza AI, Rajkumar C, Cooke J, et al. Probiotics in prevention of antibiotic-associated diarrhea: meta-analysis. BMJ 2002;324:1–6.

14. Cremonini F, Di Caro S, Nista EC, et al. Meta-analysis: the effect of probiotic administration on antibiotic-associated diarrhea. Aliment Pharmacol Ther 2002; 16:1461–7.

15. McFarland LV. Meta-analysis of probiotics for the prevention of antibiotic associated diarrhea and the treatment of clostridium difficile disease. Am J Gastroenterol 2006;101:812–22.

16. McFarland LV. Systematic review and meta-analysis of Saccharomyces boulardii in Adult Patients. World J Gastroenterol 2010;16:2202–22.

17. Duman DG, Bor S, Qzutemiz O, et al. Efficacy and safety of Saccharomyces boulardii in prevention of antibiotic-associated diarrhea due to Helicobacter pylori eradication. Eur J Gastroenterol Hepatol 2005;17:1357–61.

18. Cindoruk M, Erkan G, Karakan T, et al. Efficacy and safety of Saccharomyces boulardii in the 14-day triple anti-Helicobacter pylori therapy: a prospective randomized placebo-controlled double-blind study. Helicobacter 2007;12:309–16.

19. Cremonini F, DiCaro S, Dovino M, et al. Effect of different probiotic preparations on anti-helicobacter pylori therapy-related side effects: a parallel group, triple blind, placebo-controlled study. Am J Gastroenterol 2002;97:2744–9.

20. Videlock EJ, Cremonini F. Meta-analysis: probiotics in antibiotic-associated diarrhea. Aliment Pharmacol Ther 2012. http://dx.doi.org/10.1111/j.1365-2036.2012.05104.x.

21. Bartlett JG. Antibiotic-associated diarrhea. N Engl J Med 2002;346(5):334–8.

22. Dethlefsen L, Huse S, Sogin ML, et al. The pervasive effects of an antibiotic on the human gut microbiota, as revealed by deep 16S rRNA sequencing. PLoS Biol 2008;6(11):e280. http://dx.doi.org/10.1371/journal.pbio.0060280.

23. Caetano L, Antunes M, Han J, et al. Effect of antibiotic treatment on the intestinal metabolome. Antimicrob Agents Chemother 2011;55(4):1494–503. http://dx.doi.org/10.1128/AAC.01664-10.

24. Bartlett JG. Narrative review: the new epidemic of clostridium difficile-associated enteric disease. Ann Intern Med 2006;145:758–64.

25. Loo VG, Poirier L, Miller MA, et al. A predominant clonal multi-institutional outbreak of clostridium difficile-associated diarrhea with high morbidity and mortality. N Engl J Med 2005;353:2442–9.

26. McDonald LC, Killfore GE, Thompson A, et al. An epidemic, toxin gene-variant strain of clostridium difficile. N Engl J Med 2005;353:2433–41.

27. Riggs MM, Sethi AK, Zabarsky TF, et al. Asymptomatic arriers are a potential source for transmission of epidemic and nonepidemic Clostridium difficile strains among long-term care facility residents. Clin Infect Dis 2007;45:992.

28. Cohen SH, Gerding KN, Johnson S, et al. Clinical practice guidelines for clostridium difficile infection in adults: 2010 update by the Society for Healthcare Epidemiology of America (SHEA) and the infectious Diseases Society of America (DSA). Infect Control Hosp Epidemiol 2010;31(5):431–55.

29. Sallhamer EA, Carson K, Chang Y, et al. Fulminant Clostridium difficile Colitis. Arch Surg 2009;144(5):433–9.

30. Nelson RL, Kelsey P, Leeman H, et al. Antibiotic treatment in clostridium difficile-associated diarrhea in adults. Cochrane Database Syst Rev 2011;(9):CD004610. http://dx.doi.org/10.1002/14651858.CD004610pub4.
31. Wenisch C, Parschalk B, Hasenhundl M, et al. Comparison of vancomycin, teicoplanin, metronidazole and fusidic acid for the treatment of clostridium difficile-associated diarrhea. Clin Infect Dis 1996;22:813–8.
32. Louie TJ, Miller MA, Mullane KM, et al. Fidaxomicin versus vancomycin for clostridium difficile infection. N Engl J Med 2011;364(5):422–31.
33. Louie TJ, Peppe J, Watt CK, et al. Tolevamer, a novel nonantibiotic polymer compared with vancomycin in the treatment of mild to moderately severe Clostridium dificile associated diarrhea. Clin Infect Dis 2006;43:411–20.
34. Kelly CP, LaMont JT. Clostridium difficile – more difficult than ever. N Engl J Med 2008;359:1932–40.
35. Persky SE, Brandt L. Treatment of recurrent clostridium difficile-associated diarrhea by administration of donated stool directly through a colonoscope. Am J Gastroenterol 2000;95:3283–5.
36. Cohen SH, Gerding DN, Johnson S, et al. Clinical practice guidelines for clostridium difficile infection in adults: 2010 update by the Society for Healthcare Epidemiology of America (SHEA) and the infectious Diseases Society of America (IDSA). Infect Control Hosp Epidemiol 2010;31(5):431–55.
37. Lowy I, Molrine DC, Leav BA, et al. Treatment with monoclonal antibodies against clostridium difficile toxins. N Engl J Med 2010;362:197–205.
38. Leung DY, Kelly CP, Boguniewicz M, et al. Treatment with intravenously administered gamma globulin of chronic relapsing colitis induced by Clostridium difficile toxin. J Pediatr 1991;118:633–7.
39. Sougioultzis S, Kyne L, Drudy D, et al. Clostridium difficile toxoid vaccine in recurrent C. difficile-associated diarrhea. Gastroenterology 2005;128:764–70.
40. Aas J, Gessert CE, Bakken JS. Recurrent clostridium difficile colitis: case series involving 18 patients treated with donor stool administered via a nasogastric tube. Clin Infect Dis 2003;36:580–5.
41. Oughton MT, Loo VG, Dendukuri N, et al. Hand hygiene with soap and water is superior to alcohol rub and antiseptic wipes for removal of clostridium difficile. Infect Control Hosp Epidemiol 2009;30:939–44.
42. Stevens V, Dumyata G, Fine LS, et al. Cumulative antibiotic exposures over time and the risk of clostridium difficile infection. Clin Infect Dis 2011;53:42.
43. Valiquette L, Cossette B, Garant LP, et al. Impact of a reduction in the use of high risk antibiotics in the course of an epidemic of clostridium difficile-associated disease caused by the hyper virulent NAP1/027 strain. Clin Infect Dis 2007; 45(Suppl 2):S112–21.
44. Plummer S, Weaver MA, Harris JC, et al. Clostridium difficile pilot study: effects of probiotic supplementation in the incidence of C. difficile diarrhea. Int Microbiol 2004;7:59–62.
45. Surawicz CM, McFarland LV, Greenberg RN, et al. The search for a better treatment for recurrent clostridium difficile disease: use of high-dose vancomycin combined with Saccharomyces boulardii. Clin Infect Dis 2000;31: 1012–7.
46. Boyle RJ, Robins-Browne RM, Tank Mimi LK. Probiotic use in clinical practice: what are the risks? Am J Clin Nutr 2006;83:1256–64.
47. Pakyz A, Carroll NV, Harpe SE, et al. Economic impact of Clostridium difficile infection in a multihospital cohort of academic health centers. Pharmacotherapy 2011;31(6):546–51.

48. McGlone SM, Bailey RR, Zimmer SM, et al. The economic burden of clostridium difficile. Clin Microbiol Infect 2012;18(3):282–9.
49. Musa S, Thomson S, Cowan M, et al. Clostridium difficile infection and inflammatory bowel disease. Scand J Gastroenterol 2010;45(3):261–72.
50. Kelsen JR, Kim J, Latta D, et al. Recurrence rate of clostridium difficile infection in hospitalized pediatric patients with inflammatory bowel disease. Inflamm Bowel Dis 2011;17(1):50–5.
51. Hempel S, Newberry SJ, Maher AR, et al. Probiotics for the prevention and treatment of antibiotic-associated diarrhea. JAMA 2012;307(18):1959–69.

Fecal Microbiota Transplantation
Techniques, Applications, and Issues

Thomas Julius Borody, MD, PhD, Jordana Campbell, BSc*

KEYWORDS

- Fecal microbiota transplantation • *Clostridium difficile* • Ulcerative colitis
- Probiotics • Microbiome • Microbiota

KEY POINTS

- Fecal microbiota transplantation (FMT) is now arguably the most effective form of *Clostridium difficile* eradication, consistently achieving cure rates of greater than 90% in patients by numerous investigators.
- The therapy's success in *C difficile* infection (CDI) colitis indicates the potential value of FMT in idiopathic ulcerative colitis (UC).
- The authors' group treated the first UC patient in May 1988, which resulted in a durable clinical and histologic cure, suggesting a cure for UC is possible.
- It is the authors' current clinical impression that although *C difficile* is easily eradicated with a single FMT infusion, multiple and recurrent infusions are required to achieve prolonged remission or cure in UC.
- Manipulation of the colonic microbiota represents an exciting therapeutic strategy in several conditions where the gut microbiota has been implicated, including UC, as well as previously unexpected applications, such as obesity, diabetes, and several neurologic disorders.

DESCRIPTION AND HISTORY OF FMT

FMT is the currently accepted term to describe the "infusion of a fecal suspension from a healthy individual into the gastrointestinal tract of an individual with colonic disease."[1–7] Although the notion of FMT is at first unpalatable and inconceivable to some, the concept has existed for many decades and has been used successfully

Thomas J. Borody has a pecuniary interest in the Centre for Digestive Diseases, where fecal microbiota transplantation is a treatment option for patients and has filed patents in this area; Jordana Campbell has no financial interest or affiliation with any institution, organization, or company relating to the article.

No support or funding, including pharmaceutical and industry support, was received for work undertaken relating to the manuscript.

Centre for Digestive Diseases, Level 1, 229 Great North Road, Five Dock, New South Wales 2046, Australia

* Corresponding author.

E-mail address: jordana.campbell@cdd.com.au

Gastroenterol Clin N Am 41 (2012) 781–803
http://dx.doi.org/10.1016/j.gtc.2012.08.008
0889-8553/12/$ – see front matter © 2012 Elsevier Inc. All rights reserved.

clinically. Historically, the first recorded case of enteric flora transplantation was described by the Italian anatomist, Fabricius Acquapendente, in the seventeenth century, when he reported, "I have heard of animals which lost the capacity to ruminate, which, when one puts into their mouth a portion of the materials from the mouth of another ruminant which that animal has already chewed, they immediately start chewing and recover their former health."[8] Since that time, transfaunation has been used in veterinary practice for cattle, horses, sheep, and various other animals suffering from rumination disorders and colitis.[3–5] The first recorded use in humans dates back more than 50 years to its use for antibiotic-induced staphylococcal pseudomembranous colitis (PMC),[9,10] where it resulted in rapid recovery of previously moribund patients. In the face of the rapidly worsening current CDI epidemic, this therapy has shown great promise as an inexpensive, safe, and highly efficient treatment for recurrent and refractory CDI, which achieves results current pharmaceuticals cannot achieve.

The first published case of FMT in humans was by Eiseman and colleagues[9] in 1958, when they reported the successful treatment of 4 patients with severe PMC using fecal enemas (**Table 1**). At the time, the investigators were unaware they were treating CDI because *C difficile* was not recognized as a cause of PMC until 1978. Three of 4 patients were suffering with life-threatening fulminant PMC, which then carried a 75% mortality rate. The patients had failed all available therapies and in desperation the physicians resorted to fecal retention enemas, which resulted in prompt recovery of all patients and facilitated their discharge from hospital within days. At the time, the investigators expressed their hope that a "more complete evaluation of this simple therapeutic measure can be given further clinical trial by others."

Since FMT's first introduction into medical practice in 1958, more than 500 patients have been treated for CDI in 35 publications with a cumulative cure rate of 95%.[5,9–41] The results are summarized in **Table 2**. At the authors' center alone, approximately 100 patients have been treated for CDI, spanning 24 years.

FMT BROUGHT INTO CLINICAL USE AFTER THE CDI EPIDEMIC

Since 2000, there has been a steady increase in CDI rates in numerous health care facilities in the United States, Canada, and Europe, and CDI has reached epidemic proportions in the United States due in part to the emergence of the new hypervirulent toxigenic strains, such as the NAP1/BI/027 strain. This strain has increased toxins A and B production and high-level resistance to fluoroquinolones, secretes an additional binary toxin, and is associated with increased disease severity and worsening outcomes. It has been implicated in outbreaks of CDI worldwide and isolated from 82% of CDI cases during the 2001 to 2003 Quebec outbreaks, where hundreds of patients were infected and several deaths occurred,[43] as well as the devastating outbreak in the Niagara, Ontario, area that caused more than 30 deaths in 2011.[44]

An estimated 3 million new acute CDIs are diagnosed annually in the United States alone.[45] Of these 3 million cases, up to 35%, or approximately 1.05 million patients, fail initial antibiotic treatment and experience a symptomatic relapse.[46] Of this relapsing population, approximately 50% to 65% of patients go on to have multiple relapses (MR-CDI).[47] More worrying is the subset of acute CDI patients who progress to severe CDI due to antibiotic nonresponse, particularly in the presence of the hypervirulent 027 strain[48] and, from there, fulminant CDI (F-CDI), which is frequently fatal.

The rapidly changing epidemiology of CDI in recent years has largely caught the medical community off-guard, and the response has been generally ineffective. Strategies to counter this epidemic included discontinuing the inciting antibiotic and

Table 1
Summary of cases from Eiseman and colleagues

Case	Precipitating Events	Symptoms	Failed Therapies	Response to FMT
Case 1	Gastrectomy. Mixed antibiotic regimen postoperatively.	"Appeared to be in the terminal stages of his critical illness." Abdominal distention, vomiting, bloody diarrhea, marked hypotension.	Vasopressors, hydrocortisone, fluid therapy, albamycin	1 d Post-FMT: marked improvement in condition, bloody diarrhea ceased.
Case 2	Subtotal gastrectomy. Achromycin postoperatively	"Desperately ill" with PMC. Frequent loose, mucoid, greenish bowel movements. On fourth postoperative day—"profound shock appeared moribund."	Hydrocortisone, erythromycin, albamycin, lactobacillus	Diarrhea stopped within 48 h of FMT, "clinical response to fecal enemas was dramatic with disappearance of diarrhea."
Case 3	Preoperative sulfasuxidine and neomycin. Postoperative achromycin, penicillin and streptomycin.	After left hemicolectomy profuse watery diarrhea and fever.		48 h Post-FMT diarrhea completely ceased. Discharged 5 d later.
Case 4	Achromycin for sinusitis	Suddenly developed "severe and life-threatening" profuse watery and bloody diarrhea with fever.	IV fluid and electrolyte replacement. Intramuscular chloromycetin.	Within 24 h diarrhea had ceased. Patient made an "uneventful recovery."

Data from Eiseman B, Silen W, Bascom GS, et al. Fecal enema as an adjunct in the treatment of pseudomembranous enterocolitis. Surgery 1958;44:854–9.

Table 2
Published reports of FMT in CDI

Study	Indication	No. of Patients	Mode of Administration	Outcome
Eiseman et al,[9] 1958	Severe PMC	4	Fecal enema	Dramatic resolution of PMC in all patients (100%)
Cutolo et al,[10] 1959	PMC	1	Cantor tube, then fecal enema	Resolution
Fenton et al,[11] 1974	PMC	1	Fecal enema	Symptom resolution within 24 h; sigmoidoscopy at 4 d revealed normal mucosa.
Bowden et al,[12] 1981	PMC	16	Fecal enema (n = 15); enteric tube (n = 1)	Rapid/dramatic response in 13/20 (65%). 3/20 (15%) patients died; no PMC on autopsy in 2 the third patient had small-bowel PMC.
Schwan et al,[13] 1984	Relapsing CDI	1	Fecal enema	Prompt/complete normalization of bowel function.
Tvede and Rask-Madsen,[14] 1989	Relapsing CDI	6	Fecal enema	Prompt C difficile eradication and symptom resolution. Normal bowel function within 24 h.
Flotterod and Hopen,[15] 1991	Refractory CDI	1	Duodenal tube	C difficile eradication
Paterson et al,[16] 1994	Chronic CDI	7	Colonoscope	Rapid symptom relief. Resolution in all (100%).
Harkonen,[17] 1996	PMC	1	Colonoscope	Diarrhea ceased immediately and symptoms had not recurred by 8 mo post FMT.
Lund-Tonneson et al,[18] 1998	CDI	18	Colonoscope (n = 17); gastrostoma (n = 1)	15/18 (83.3%) Clinically cured post-FMT without relapse
Persky and Brandt,[19] 2000	Recurrent CDI	1	Colonoscope	Immediate symptom resolution; C difficile eradication persisted at 5-year follow-up.
Faust et al,[20] 2002	Recurrent PMC	6	Unknown	All patients (100%) clinically cured postinfusion.
Aas et al,[21] 2003	Recurrent C difficile colitis	18	Nasogastric tube	15/18 (83.3%) Cured; 2 (11.1%) patients died of unrelated illnesses; 1 treatment failure (5.5%).
Borody et al,[5] 2003	Chronic CDI	24	Colonoscope and/or rectal enema and/or nasojejunal tube	Eradicated CDI in 20/24 patients (83.3%) with negative toxins and stool culture.

Reference	Diagnosis	N	Route	Outcome
Jorup-Rönström et al,[22] 2006	Recurrent CDI	5	Fecal enema	All (100%) patients clinically asymptomatic post-FMT.
Wettstein et al,[23] 2007	Relapsing CDI	16	Colonoscope (day 1), then enemas 5, 10, or 24 d.	Eradication of CDI in 15/16 pts (93.8%), confirmed via negative culture or toxin assay.
Louie et al,[24] 2008	Relapsing CDI	45	Rectal catheter	CDI resolved in 43/45 (95.6%) patients.
Niewdorp et al,[25] 2008	Recurrent CDI	7 (2 of Whom with the 027 strain)	Jejunal infusion via duodenal catheter	C difficile eradication in all patients (100%), confirmed via culture and/or toxin assay.
You et al,[26] 2008	F-CDI	1	Fecal enema	Bowel function, BP, and leukocytosis normalized; oliguria resolved, and both vasopressin and venous hemofiltration were discontinued.
Hellemans et al,[27] 2009	CDI	1	Colonoscope	C difficile eradication
MacChonachie et al,[28] 2009	Recurrent CDI	15	Nasogastric tube	13/15 (86.7%) Asymptomatic post-FMT.
Arkkila et al,[29] 2010	Recurrent CDI	37 (11 of whom with the 027 strain)	Colonoscope	C difficile eradication in 34/37(92%) patients.
Khoruts et al,[30] 2010	Recurrent CDI	1	Colonoscope	C difficile eradicated, confirmed via negative culture. Remained negative at 6-month follow-up.
Yoon and Brandt,[31] 2010	Recurrent CDI/PMC	12, 2 of whom had PMC	Colonoscope	12/12 (100%) Exhibited durable clinical response.
Rohlke et al,[32] 2010	Recurrent CDI	19	Colonoscope	18/19 (94.7%) Clinically asymptomatic between 6 mo and 5 y post-FMT.
Silverman et al,[33] 2010	Chronic recurrent CDI	7	Low-volume fecal enema	All (100%) patients clinically asymptomatic.
Garborg et al,[34] 2010	Recurrent CDI	40	Colonoscopic = 2; transduodenal = 38	Eradication of C difficile in 33/40 patients (82.5%).
Russel et al,[35] 2010	Relapsing CDI	1	Nasogastric tube	Resolved diarrhea by 36 h. C difficile toxin negative.
Kelly and De Leon,[36] 2010	Chronic recurrent CDI	12	Colonoscope	All (100%) patients exhibited clinical response.

(continued on next page)

Table 2
(continued)

Study	Indication	No. of Patients	Mode of Administration	Outcome
Mellow and Kanatzar,[37] 2010	Recurrent and refractory CDI	13	Colonoscope	12/13 (92.3%) *C difficile* toxin negative with rapid resolution of diarrhea.
Kassam et al,[38] 2010	CDI	14	Fecal enema	All (100%) patients complete clinical resolution.
Kelly et al,[39] 2012	Relapsing CDI	26	Colonoscope	24/26 Cured of CDI with resolution of diarrhea.
Hamilton et al,[40] 2012	Recurrent CDI	43	Colonoscope	86% Eradication rate (37/43) by symptom resolution/negative PCR testing for CDI toxin.
Mattila et al,[41] 2012	Refractory CDI	70	Colonoscope	66/70 Recovered (94%) *C difficile* eradicated.
Brandt et al,[42] 2012	Recurrent CDI	77	Colonoscope	Primary cure rate of 91%. Secondary cure rate of 98%. Resolution of diarrhea in 74% of patients by day 3.

Abbreviation: CDAD, *C difficile*–associated diarrhea.

restricting the use of high-risk antibiotics and use of specific antibiotic treatments once the etiology was known. These interventions, however, have failed to arrest the epidemic and, in retrospect, have not taken into account the pathophysiology of relapsing CDI. Despite CDI most commonly occurring after antibiotic exposure, first-line therapies rely heavily on antibiotics, such as vancomycin, metronidazole, and fidaxomicin, which fail to correct the underlying flora deficiencies. Once patients have failed first-line therapies, current CDI therapies lack a solution for the underlying bowel flora deficiencies driving the MR-CDI.

The inability of antibiotic-based measures to hinder the spread of infection suggests that unless drastic and novel therapeutic strategies are used that address the underlying microbiota defects, this epidemic will continue to spread unabated. The predictable consequences include rising morbidity, prolonged illness, greater risk of complications, and higher mortality rates. A crisis has been building in the past 2 decades due in part to the emerging epidemic strain and reducing efficacy of antibiotics, particularly in the face of the epidemic strains. Instead of predicting and preparing for this day by focusing on the cause, however, the medical community has continued to rely on antibiotics, incorporating new models,[49] sophisticated combinations,[50] and novel routes of administrations[51]; reducing vancomycin protocols[52]; and developing antitoxin antibodies.[53] An alternative and more effective approach is to address the fundamental microbiota pathology[30]—known since 1989.[14] The industry is scrambling to develop new therapeutic strategies, such as toxin scavengers, immune stimulants, and newer antimicrobials, to counteract this epidemic rather than repairing the underlying microbiota defect. These therapies will unlikely be available for several years, leaving prescribing physicians limited in their choice of curative options while prolonging the duration of the epidemic. It is not hard to fully grasp this scenario, which demands focus and action to avert an ongoing global CDI health care crisis, the latest casualty being Australia with the start of its epidemic.[54–56]

FMT offers the particularly attractive therapeutic solution of eradicating CDI through the re-establishment of normal intestinal flora composition via the implantation of missing fecal components provided from a healthy donor.[57] Originally a last-ditch therapy for dying patients,[9–11] the nearly 100% cure rates achieved in MR-CDI and F-CDI have driven institutions worldwide to adopt FMT earlier with an emphasis for FMT to become the first-line treatment option.[58]

GUT MIROBIOTA—THE VIRTUAL ORGAN

The *human gut microbiota* is the term used to collectively describe the complex ecosystem of some 10^{14} bacterial cells housed within the gastrointestinal tract.[59] Extensively more complex than previously believed,[60] the number of microbial cells outnumber the human somatic cells by approximately 1 order of magnitude. Concurrently the microbiome, which is the collective genomes of the gut microbiota, outweighs the human genome by up to 2 orders of magnitude.[61] Recent research has offered new insights into the microbial diversity of the gut microbiota, with the dominant organisms belonging to 7 main bacterial divisions (ie, Firmicutes, Bacteroides, Proteobacteria, Fusobacteria, Verrucomicrobia, Cyanobacteria, and Actinobacteria). Of these, Firmicutes and Bacteroides are the most abundant of the species, comprising approximately 70% of all gut bacteria.[62]

Until recently, the function of the gut microbiota has been underestimated. Commonly believed a waste product of digestion destined for elimination, rarely was it considered an organ of microbial cells contained within humans with critical roles in immunity and energy metabolism—among other roles. With the development of molecular-based metagenomics, metabolomics, and proteomics,[62] various functions of the gastrointestinal microbiota are beginning to be unraveled. Several diverse functions can be ascribed to this microbial organ, summarized in 4 broad categories: (1) pathogen resistance and clearance, (2) immunomodulation, (3) control of epithelial cell proliferation and differentiation, and (4) nutrition and metabolism.

Constantly interfacing with the external environment, arguably one of the most important functions of the gut microbiota, is defense against invading pathogens. This occurs not only through competition for nutrients and adhesion sites, termed *colonization resistance*,[63] but also through the production of bacteriocins and bacterial-derived immunomodulatory molecules. The intestinal microbiota has been identified as a rich source of protective probiotics, which produce novel antimicrobial and, more specifically, antipathogenic bacteriocins. Thuricin CD is a narrow-spectrum bacteriocin produced by *Bacillus thuringiensis* found to possess potent activity against *C difficile*. For the most part—similar to bacterially derived vancomycin[64]—bacteriocins have a narrow spectrum of activity, inhibiting strains closely related to the producer. Some bacteriocins, however, such as nisin, possess a broad spectrum of inhibition, active against a vast array of gram-positive bacteria.[65] In recent years, there has been a particular focus on bacteriocin-producing gut bacteria. Bacteriocin production is believed to provide strains with a competitive advantage within complex microbial environments as a consequence of their associated antimicrobial activity, enabling the establishment and prevalence of producing strains as well as directly inhibiting pathogens within the gut. The production of these antimicrobial peptides and associated intestinal producing strains is one likely mechanism contributing to FMT's efficacy to beneficially influence the microbial communities of the gastrointestinal tract and facilitate durable implantation.[57]

RATIONALE FOR FMT USE

Depletion in intestinal microbiota constituents, including Bacteroidetes and Firmicutes phyla, have been demonstrated in patients with initial or recurrent *C difficile* infection[14,30] and seems to be associated, or perhaps causal, in several other conditions.[60] The rationale behind FMT includes the reintroduction of a complete, stable community of gut microorganisms aimed at repairing or replacing the disrupted native microbiota to correct the underlying imbalance. It is presumed this microbiota repair eradicates or hinders pathogens, which may be causing the targeted condition (eg, CDI). The current application of probiotics at best aims to alter the metabolic or immunologic activity of the residing native gut microbiota. A cultured single or few strains, which exist in low numbers and struggle to implant onto the bowel epithelium. FMT results in a durable, long-term implantation of donor flora.[57] In one report by Khoruts and colleagues,[30] transplantation of fecal microbiota from a healthy individual into a recipient with recurrent CDI resulted in resolution of symptoms and a fecal bacterial composition dominated by *Bacteroides* spp and an uncharacterized butyrate producing bacterium, which closely matched those of the healthy donor. Implantation of members of the *Bifidobacterium* genus, the *Bacteroides* and *Clostridium coccoides* groups, and the *Clostridium leptum* subgroup, has further been demonstrated after transplantation of donor stool for up to 24 weeks.[57] These studies suggest that long-term restoration of the disrupted gut microbiota by fecal transplantation is achievable. Hence, FMT is likely not only to repair the depleted flora but also introduce species whose bacteriocins may eradicate susceptible pathogens with these antibiotic-like molecules and presumably restore the multiple functions of microbiota (enumerated previously).

TORY BOWEL DISEASE

e gut microbiota in the pathogenesis of inflammatory bowel disease shed. Many studies have reported marked alterations in fecal and communities in IBD patients versus healthy controls, with several decreased abundance of dominant commensal members, such nd IV groups, *Bacteroides*, and *Bifidobacteria*, and also a concom- trimental bacteria, such as sulfate-reducing bacteria, *Escherichia* re, some patients with Crohn disease have been shown to have *Faecalibacterium prausnitzii* in mucosa-associated microbiota.[68] ı—a prevalent Firmicutes species and an important butyrate metabolites that reduce proinflammatory cytokine production, IL)-12 and interferon-γ; increases production of IL-10; and inhibits tis in a mouse model. Qin and colleagues[60] demonstrated low diver- ə of microbiota abnormality in UC and Crohn disease.

that an infective agent or agents could reduce diversity. Infection ave been shown to alter the composition of the intestinal micro- ways. Lupp and colleagues,[69] in a murine model of enterohaemor- ction, showed that *Citrobacter rodentium* infection drastically ers of colonic microbiota and extensively altered the composition crobiota. Similarly, Barman and colleagues,[70] in a murine model of rium infection, reported a 95% decrease in total bacterial number arge intestine of mice after *S typhimurium* infection (Borody TJ, M, et al, personal communication, 2011). In addition, alterations osition preceded the onset of diarrhea, suggesting the involvement ensal interactions and/or host responses unrelated to diarrhea.

an exhaustive review of reported microbiota abnormalities in IBD; ce has tipped in favor of the instrumental role that abnormal micro- causality. This concept supersedes the older Podolsky theory, ımmatory bowel disease is thought to result from inappropriate tion of the mucosal immune system driven by the presence of a."[71] An infectious cause has long been proposed for IBD but ıe complexity of the normal flora been better appreciated, which ' difficult it would be to identify certain scarce pathogens among ıers of flora components. Known infective agents, such a *Campylo-* ı *E coli*, often result in a visible colitis, which heals after the causal he colon.[72] CDI colitis also heals after successful eradication with of CDI colitis with FMT in part drove the authors' FMT studies in ' rationale was that if *C difficile* can cause colitis and FMT can ' treatment should be applied to IBD. This seemed to work in the authors treated their first UC patient in 1988 with others d detailed long-term follow-up in 6 cases reported in 2003.[5] Today, ears later, that first patient remains asymptomatic and in histologic

rketed therapies and lends further credence to an infective cause, disprov-
viously accepted theory of an "aberrant reaction to normal colonic flora."[71]
erhaps be one of the great breakthroughs in modern medicine and involves
id accepting an entirely new concept involving a close co-existance with
a. If UC can be cured by infusing "normal colonic flora" from a healthy indi-
the colon of a patient with UC, accepted etiologic dogma needs to be
and rejected. Unlike even recalcitrant CDI, however, in which a single
T is sufficient to eradicate the infection,[58] the abnormal microbial commu-
)—luminal as well as intramucosal[74]—are resistant to change, requiring not
recurrent, administration of scheduled infusions.[2] It is this discovery of the
ipeated infusions of normal flora that reverses inflammation in most cases
en medically unresponsive colitis (ulcerative and Crohn) and also gives
) the mechanism of inflammation at the mucosal interface. Examples of
itive cases of IBD reversal with FMT alone are shown in **Figs. 1–5**.

-old patient with a 10-year history of severe UC, uncontrolled with anti-
)ry agents, steroids, antibiotics, and finally anti–tumor necrosis factor
iderwent FMT. Pre-FMT symptoms included severe diarrhea with marked
nd presence of blood and mucus. The patient underwent colonoscopy
first FMT was administered. After this, daily rectal infusions were performed
followed by 26 weekly rectal infusions. The patient experienced an imme-
iction in symptoms, passing 2 formed stools daily without blood, urgency,
Follow-up colonoscopy at 12 months revealed virtually nil inflammation
iand she remains clinically well at 12 months on no medication.

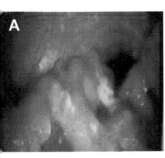
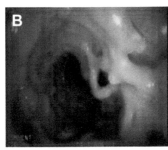

Pre-FMT: edema while on numerous combined therapies. (*B*) Pre-FMT: extensive
)s.

with a 5-year history of UC/Crohn disease, ultimately failing immu-
ntibiotics, and anti–tumor necrosis factor therapy, underwent FMT.
d anal fissures, severe abdominal pain, and bloody diarrhea up to
ily, and colectomy had been advised. Patient commenced daily
is for 2 months, followed by infusions of ever lessening frequency.
MT, rectal bleeding had resolved, and diarrhea had ceased at
o colonoscopy revealed no inflammation with some residual pseu-
ht colon.

B

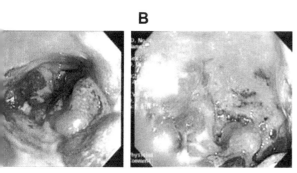

severe luminal inflammatory changes initially. (*B*) Post-FMT.

B

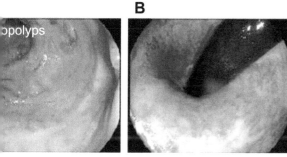

some pseudopolyps in the ascending colon at 9 months. (*B*) Post-FMT:
showing return of vasculature.

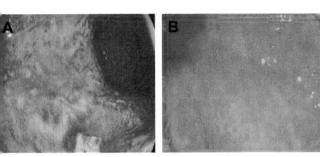

e-FMT: figure rectal inflammation before FMT. (*B*) Post-FMT: normal mucosa in
ith no signs of protitis.

GING APPLICATIONS

CDI epidemic, coupled with the burgeoning interest in the gut microbiota,
e recent resurgence of FMT as a powerful clinical therapy for CDI (**Fig. 6**).
t is fortuitous that the CDI epidemic facilitated the use of FMT to other
inal conditions. Andrews and colleagues[2] in the authors' group treated
with chronic, severe constipation using FMT and reported a substantial
it in 89% (40/45) of these patients, with improved defecation and resolu-
ing and abdominal pain. Of the 30 patients contacted at long-term follow-
onths), 18 (60%) continued to report normal defecation without laxative
eparate report of a constipated patient, both anorectal dysmotility and

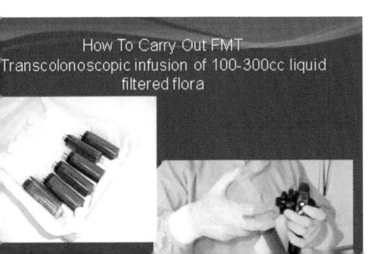

How To Carry Out FMT
Transcolonoscopic infusion of 100-300cc liquid
filtered flora

deep pseudomelanosis coli were reversed after FMT.[75] Borody and colleagues,[73] in a case series of 55 patients with irritable bowel syndrome (IBS) and IBD treated with FMT, reported that 36% (20/55) patients were deemed cured post-FMT and 16% (9/55) patients reported a decrease in symptoms. Such clinical documentations open the door to a better understanding of the profound contribution abnormal microbiota plays in IBD and IBS and perhaps to channelling scarce funding into microbiota research both in the diagnostic and therapeutic fields.

There is also compelling evidence that the importance of the intestinal microbiota extends beyond the intestine. Several studies during the past decade have implicated the intestinal microbiota in the pathogenesis of several disorders, including obesity,[76] diabetes,[77] autism,[78] myasthenia gravis,[79] rheumatoid arthritis,[80] and other conditions. The metabolic syndrome epidemic, associated with obesity and related health problems, is arguably the greatest single health care challenge in the industrialized world, rapidly spreading to encompass less developed nations. Energy metabolism is a well-recognized primary function of the gut microbiota. Differences in distal gut microbiota composition have been reported in human studies and mice models of obesity, with a shift in the ratio of Firmicutes and Bacteroidetes.[81,82] Ley and colleagues,[82] analyzing 5088 bacterial 16S rRNA gene sequences, reported that *ob/ob* animals have a 50% reduction in the abundance of Bacteroidetes and a proportional increase in Firmicutes. Turnbaugh and colleagues,[76] transplanting lean and obese cecal microbiotas into germ-free wild-type mouse recipients, demonstrated that colonization of germ-free mice with an obese microbiota results in a significantly greater increase in total body fat than colonization with a lean microbiota and that this trait is transmissible. In 2010, Vrieze and colleagues[83] reported the results of a double-blind, randomized controlled trial of FMT in 18 men with the metabolic syndrome. Fifty percent of patients received fecal material from lean male donors and the other 50% were implanted with their own feces as controls. Transplantation from lean donors resulted in a marked reduction of fasting triglyceride levels in patients with the metabolic syndrome. No effect was observed in the control group reinfusing their own feces. In addition, peripheral and hepatic insulin sensitivity markedly improved after 6 weeks in the lean donor group. This was again not observed in the control group. These findings suggest that intentional manipulation of community structure may be useful for regulating energy balance in obese individuals.

Along similar lines, the gut microbiota has been hypothesized as playing a role in the pathophysiology of eating disorders. Armougon and colleagues,[81] analyzing the gut microbiota of individuals with anorexia nervosa, found increased levels of the methanogen *Methanobrevibacter smithii* in the anorexic patient population versus controls. At the authors' clinic, 2 patients were treated with repeated home FMT for their IBS and coexisting anorexia nervosa, and both regained an interest in food and subsequently regained weight, one of them dramatically.

Several neurologic conditions have associated bowel dysfunction. Up to 80% of patients with Parkinson disease report constipation as an early symptom that can precede the onset of motor symptoms by up to 2 decades.[84] In addition, men who experience less than 1 bowel movement daily have a 4-fold increase of developing Parkinson disease in later life.[85] In 2009, the authors reported a 73-year-old man with chronic constipation who was treated with vancomycin, colchicine (Colgout), and metronidazole (Flagyl) for his constipation.[86] His baseline motor symptoms included marked pillrolling hand tremor, micrographia, positive glabellar tap reflex, and cogwheel rigidity. When reviewed after 21 days on antibiotic treatment, he reported a marked improvement in his constipation symptoms, defecating daily with ease. Surprisingly, he also reported a marked improvement in his Parkinson disease symptoms, with a visible decrease in tremor commencing 10 days into therapy. At 6 and 10 months on continuous therapy, he reported resolution of neurologic symptoms, including absence of persistent tremors and glabellar tap reflex, and he lost his cogwheel rigidity. The remarkable resolution of constipation coupled with neurologic near normalization with antibiotics, one of which is not absorbed, suggest that the gut microbiota is involved in the pathogenesis of this disease. Braak and colleagues[87] postulated this from histopathologic data and suggested a microbial origin arising in the gut with brain pathology developing later.

This gut-brain connection is also clear in a case of a 28-year-old woman with myoclonic dystonia and long-standing diarrhea.[88] The movement disorder began at the same time as the diarrhea, at age 6, and progressed in severity until age 18, when they plateaued. Predominant neurologic symptoms consisted of tremors of the hands, arms, and neck and muscle spasms, including severe writers cramps, all associated with worsening diarrhea. Consultation with several neurologists confirmed the diagnosis of myoclonic dystonia. Gastrointestinal symptoms included frequent diarrhea with daily loose motions (up to 10 per day), bloating, flatulence, and fatigue. Treatment of a presumed pathogen was initiated with vancomycin, rifaximin and metronidazole (Flagyl) for her diarrheal symptoms, which resulted in rapid improvement in diarrhea and gradual but then profound improvement in her movement disorder of 90% to where she could write continuously in excess of 5 minutes, carry mugs of coffee, and eat with a fork. At baseline, the patient could not write for more than 30 seconds, could not hold cups without dropping them, and could not use a knife and fork due to her symptoms.

Other gut-brain influence examples include the virtually complete and prolonged (>15 years) normalization of previously documented severe multiple sclerosis (MS) symptoms in 3 patients who underwent FMT for constipation.[3] Such exceptional observations point to the potential role of the gut microbiota in promoting the pathologic inflammation that underlies MS. Using a mouse model of MS, Mazmanian and colleagues[89] showed that the presence of segmented filamentous bacteria in the gut plays a central role in the development of experimental autoimmune encephalomyelitis through induction of Th17 cells and consequential IL-17 production in the gut and spinal cord. The association of elevated levels of IL-17 with MS is well established. Targeting the source of the autoimmune response (gut microbes) rather than the end result (elevated levels of IL-17) may be a valid approach to treating some cases of MS.

Several studies have described increased prevalence of gastrointestinal dysfunction and histologic changes in the gastrointestinal tract of autistic children versus healthy controls, with overgrowth of certain bacterial species or other changes in the gut microbiota frequently reported.[90,91] In 1971, Goodwin and colleagues[92] were among the first to make this observation, reporting on 15 autistic patients, 6 of whom had bulky, odorous, loose, or diarrheal stools. Horvath and Perman[93] confirmed these findings in 2002 when they revealed a high prevalence of gastrointestinal dysfunction in 412 autistic children surveyed over a 6-year period from 1996 to 2002. The results reported that 84.1% of autistic patients had at least 1 gastrointestinal symptom comprising diarrhea, constipation, foul-smelling stools, abdominal discomfort, bloating, belching, or reflux versus only 31.2% of healthy siblings ($P<.0001$). Valicenti-McDermott and colleagues,[94] comparing the prevalence of gut symptoms in autistic children versus developmentally disabled children and those with normal development in a cross-sectional study, found a history of gastrointestinal symptoms in 70% of children with ASD compared with 28% of children with typical development ($P<.001$) and 42% of children with DD.

Alterations in gut *Clostridium* species are commonly detected in autism. Finegold and colleagues,[90] comparing fecal flora from children with regressive autism versus controls, found significantly higher *Clostridial* counts in autistic group. Additionally, the number of *Clostridial* species was much greater in the autistic group versus controls. Furthermore, 9 species of *Clostridium* were found in autistic children that were not found in controls. In a later study, Song and colleagues[95] found statistically significant cell count differences between autistic and control children for *C bolteae* and clusters I and XI of the *Clostridium* groups. Mean counts of *C bolteae* and clusters I and XI in autistic children were 46-fold ($P = .01$), 9-fold ($P = .014$), and 3.5-fold ($P = .004$) greater than those in control children, respectively.

Parracho and colleagues[78] surveying 58 ASD children and healthy controls not only found an overwhelming prevalence of gastrointestinal disorders in autism (91.4% vs 25% in siblings and 0% in unrelated healthy children ($P<.05$)) but also markedly increased levels of *C histolyticum* in the ASD groups compared with healthy unrelated children and healthy siblings ($P<.01$ and $P<.05$, respectively). In another study, Finegold's group detected *Desulfovibrio* bacteria specifically in the autistic group but not in the control group also susceptible to vancomycin.[91] If *Clostridia* and *Desulfovibrios* contribute etiologically, treatment with oral vancomycin, which targets both species and has poor systemic absorption, should lead to significant improvement in these patients. This was the case when Sandler and colleagues[96] treating a 4.5-year-old boy with autism and chronic diarrhea with vancomycin, reported dramatic results. The child had displayed normal motor, cognitive, and social development until the age of 18 months, when he received recurrent antibiotic treatments for otitis media and subsequently developed diarrhea with gradual decline in motor cognitive and social development. A 12-week therapeutic trial of vancomycin (125 mg 4 times per day) was initiated, which resulted in a rapid and significant clinical improvement. The child became affectionate and calm and promptly achieved toilet training and increased vocabulary. Follow-up behavioral assessments revealed an increase in on-task performance, compliance, and parental requests; awareness of environmental surrounds; and persistence when engaging in positive activities. After discontinuation of vancomycin therapy, behavioral deterioration was observed and although still improved over baseline, he eventually lost most of the gains. A follow-up study of 10 autistic children treated with oral vancomycin resulted in a short-term benefit in 8 of 10 patients.[96] Efficacy was largely lost, however, after stopping vancomycin.

For many years, we have highlighted the brain-gut axis, especially in relation to functional bowel disorders, but much of this work has previously been focused on a top-down approach. New work involving the gut microbiota indicate that this communication network is bidirectional and that events occurring in the gut microbiota, not just the gut enteric nervous system, also can have an impact on the function of the central nervous system (CNS). Research has shown that this communication likely occurs via the vagus nerve.[97] Examples include work by Bravo and colleagues,[98] who demonstrated that *Lactobacillus rhamnosus* can modulate behavior and CNS biochemistry in healthy mice via the vagus nerve. Similarly McLean and colleagues[99] previously showed that *Bifidobacterium longum* (Bl NCC3001) normalizes behavior and CNS biochemistry in mice with mild colitis, also mediated via the vagus nerve. Several pathogens, however, also exploit this link. The vagus nerve provides the route of ascent to the CNS for transporting tetanus neurotoxin.[100] Prion infections (including Creutzfeldt-Jakob disease in humans, bovine spongiform encephalopathy in cattle, and scrapie in sheep) use the enteric and peripheral nervous system to reach their ultimate target of the central nervous system. The new concept should also include gut

Table 3
Donor absolute and relative exclusion criteria

Absolute Exclusion Criteria[a]	Relative Exclusion Criteria
Risk of infectious agent[a]	History of major gastrointestinal surgery (eg, gastric bypass)
Known HIV, hepatitis B or C infections	Metabolic syndrome
Known exposure to HIV or viral hepatitis within the previous 12 mo	Systemic autoimmunity (eg, MS, connective tissue disease)
High-risk sexual behaviors (eg, sexual contact with anyone with HIV/acquired immune deficiency syndrome or hepatitis; men who have sex with men; prostitution for drugs or money)	Atopic diseases, including asthma and eczema, eosinophilic disorders of the gastrointestinal tract
Use of illicit drugs	Chronic pain syndromes (eg, chronic fatigue syndrome, fibromyalgia)
Tattoo or body piercing within 6 mo	
Incarceration or history of incarceration	
Known current communicable disease (eg, upper respiratory tract infection)	
Risk factors for variant Creutzfeldt-Jacob disease	
Travel within the last 6 mo to areas of the world where diarrheal illnesses are endemic or risk of traveler's diarrhea is high	

1. Gastrointestinal comorbidities
  a. History of IBD
  b. History of IBD, idiopathic chronic constipation or chronic diarrhea
  c. History of gastrointestinal malignancy or known polyposis	

2. Factors that can or do affect the composition of the intestinal microbiota
  a. Antibiotics within the preceding 3 mo
  b. Major immunosuppressive medication (calcineurin inhibitors, exogenous glucocorticosteroids, biologic agents, and so forth)
  c. Systemic antineoplastic agents	

3. Additional recipient considerations a. Recent ingestion of a potential allergen (eg, nuts) where recipient has a known allergy to this/these agent(s).	

[a] May be appropriate to consider.
From Bakken JS, Borody TJ, Brandt LJ et al. Treating Clostridium difficile infection with fecal microbiota transplantation. Clin Gastroenterol Hepatol 2011;9:1044–9; with permission.

microbiota-brain axis but in the reverse direction. Hence, bacterially mediated autism is an example of such a mechanism.

Circulating antigen uptake from the bowel microbiota may explain the mechanism of ongoing autoimmune-like syndrome, as in an index case of idiopathic thrombocyto-penia. The authors reported prolonged remission of idiopathic thrombocytopenia after FMT targeting UC[4] and near-complete and prolonged (>15 years) normalization of previously severe MS symptoms in 3 patients who underwent FMT for constipation.[3] Often marked improvement in chronic fatigue syndrome using FMT in 34 patients for IBS symptoms may point to a similar mechanism.[101] These serendipitous results after FMT in extraintestinal conditions not previously considered to originate in gut micro-biota may be pointing to studying the gut flora to uncover the underlying pathogenesis of these disorders and likely others.

HOW IS FMT CURRENTLY PERFORMED?

Recently, a group of international infectious disease and gastroenterology specialists published formal practice guidelines for performing FMT, outlining the rationale, methods, and indications of FMT, including screening procedures (see **Table 1**), mate-rial preparation, FMT administration, and other practical pointers.[7] The investigators advise using the American Association of Blood Banks Donor History Questionnaire[102] to screen potential donors in addition to the screening procedures listed in **Table 3**.

The infusate is prepared by homogenizing stool with a diluent, such as preservative-free normal saline, in a dedicated conventional household blender until the mixture reaches a liquid slurry consistency. The mixture is then filtered to remove particulate matter. Depending on the route of delivery, the slurry can then be poured into enema bags for rectal administration or drawn up into syringes for administration through the biopsy channel of the colonoscope. Methods used to administer FMT have included fecal suspensions via nasogastric and nasoduodenal tubes,[28,103] through the colono-scope,[16] or as a retention enema.[22] No clear superiority of one method over another has yet been demonstrated. The selection of delivery method is up to the discretion of the infectious diseases specialist or the gastroenterologist and may vary with the needs and status of individual patients.

Universal precautions should be used when preparing FMT infusate, including a hood, if possible, because stool is a level 2 biohazard. Those involved with mixing and/or handling the fecal material should wear a fluid-resistant gown, gloves, and mask with goggles or eye shield. Stool should be administered as soon as possible after passage but within 24 hours and preferably within 6 hours.

HOW WILL FMT BE PERFORMED IN THE FUTURE?

As FMT development moves forward, in the foreseeable future, the authors envision the task being best conducted by a few centralized facilities, capable of filtering and process-ing the donor material and shipping it to individual providers in frozen,[40] and ultimately in a lyophilized, form as powder for various ways of administration, including encapsulated form. This form of FMT can be used in carriers, such as yogurt or favored beverages, for administration to children or in a capsule for longer treatment in IBD or IBS.

SUMMARY

In summary, use of FMT in various conditions has opened the door to better under-stand the contributing mechanisms of previously idiopathic diseases. If some of the major diseases, such as the metabolic syndrome, IBD, and some neurologic and perhaps autoimmune conditions, are causally linked to disordered microbiota, FMT in its various delivery forms can be anticipated to have a role in therapeutic gut microbiota restoration with far-reaching effects on a society-wide scale.

REFERENCES

1. Jarvis WR, Schlosser JA, Jarvis AA, et al. National point prevalence of Clostridium difficile in US health care facility inpatient. Am J Infect Control 2008;37:263–70.
2. Andrews P, Borody TJ, Shortis NP, et al. Bacteriotherapy for chronic constipation—long term follow-up. Gastroenterology 1995;108:A563.
3. Borody TJ, Leis S, Campbell J, et al. Fecal microbiota transplantation (FMT) in multiple sclerosis (MS). Am J Gastroenterol 2011;106:S352.
4. Borody TJ, Campbell J, Torres M, et al. Reversal of idiopathic thrombocytopenia purpura (ITP) with fecal microbiota transplantation (FMT). Am J Gastroenterol 2011;106:S352.
5. Borody TJ, Warren EF, Leis S, et al. Treatment of ulcerative colitis using fecal bacteriotherapy. J Clin Gastroenterol 2003;37(1):42–7.
6. Bennet JD, Brinkman M. Treatment of ulcerative colitis by implantation of normal colonic flora. Lancet 1989;1:164.
7. Bakken JS, Borody TJ, Brandt LJ, et al. Treating *Clostridium difficile* infection with fecal microbiota transplantation. Clin Gastroenterol Hepatol 2011;9:1044–9.
8. Borody TJ, Warren EF, Leis SM, et al. Bacteriotherapy using fecal flora: toying with human motions. J Clin Gastroenterol 2004;38:475–83.
9. Eiseman B, Silen W, Bascom GS, et al. Fecal enema as an adjunct in the treatment of pseudomembranous enterocolitis. Surgery 1958;44:854–9.
10. Cutolo LC, Kleppel NH, Freund RH, et al. Fecal feedings as a therapy in Staphylococcus enterocolitis. N Y State J Med 1959;59:3831–3.
11. Fenton S, Stephenson D, Weder C, et al. Pseudomembranous colitis associated with antibiotic therapy—an emerging entity. Can Med Assoc J 1974;111:1110–4.
12. Bowden TA, Mansberger AR, Lykins LE. Pseudomembranous enterocolitis: mechanism for restoring floral homeostasis. Am Surg 1981;47:178–83.
13. Schwan A, Sjölin S, Trottestam U, et al. Relapsing Clostridium difficile enterocolitis cured by rectal infusion of normal faeces. Scand J Infect Dis 1984;16:211–5.
14. Tvede M, Rask-Madsen J. Bacteriotherapy for chronic relapsing Clostridium difficile diarrhoea in six patients. Lancet 1989;1:1156–60.
15. Flotterod O, Hopen G. Refractory Clostridium difficile infection. Untraditional treatment for antibiotic-induced colitis. Tidsskr Nor Laegeforen 1991;111: 1364–5 [in Norwegian].
16. Paterson DL, Iredell J, Whitby M. Putting back the bugs: bacterial treatment relieves chronic diarrhoea. Med J Aust 1994;160:232–3.
17. Harkonen N. Recurrent pseudomembranous colitis treated with the donor feces. Duodecim 1996;112:1803–4.
18. Lund-Tonneson S, Berstad A, Schreiner A, et al. Clostridium difficile-associated diarrhoea treated with homologous feces. Tidsskr Nor Laegeforen 1998;118: 1027–30 [in Norwegian].
19. Persky SE, Brandt LJ. Treatment of recurrent Clostridium difficile-associated diarrhoea by administration of donated stool directly through a colonoscope. Am J Gastroenterol 2000;95:3283–5.
20. Faust G, Langelier D, Haddad H, et al. Treatment of recurrent pseudomembranous colitis (RPMC) with stool transplantation (ST): report of six (6) cases. Can J Gastroenterol 2002;a002.

21. Aas J, Gessert CE, Bakken JS. Recurrent *Clostridium difficile* colitis: case series involving 18 patients treated with donor stool administered via a nasogastric tube. Clin Infect Dis 2003;36:580–5.
22. Jorup-Rönström C, Hakanson A, Persoon AK. Feces culture successful therapy in Clostridium difficile diarrhoea [abstract]. Larkartidningen 2006;103:3603–5 [in Swedish].
23. Wettstein A, Borody TJ, Leis S. Fecal bacteriotherapy—an effective treatment for relapsing symptomatic Clostridium difficile infection [abstract G67]. Presented at the 15th United European Gastroenterology Week. 2007.
24. Louie TJ. Home-based fecal flora infusion to arrest multiple-recurrent Clostridium difficile infection (CDI). Presented at the 48th Interscience Conference on Antimicrobial Agents, Chemotherapy in conjunction with the Infectious Disease Society of America. 2008.
25. Niewdorp M, Van Nood E, Speelman P, et al. Treatment of recurrent Clostridium difficile-associated diarrhoea with a suspension of donor faeces. Ned Tijdschr Geneeskd 2008;152:1927–32 [in dutch].
26. You DM, Franzos MA, Holman RP. Successful treatment of fulminant Clostridium difficile infection with fecal bacteriotherapy. Ann Intern Med 2008; 148:632–3.
27. Hellemans R, Naegels S, Holvoet J. Faecal transplantation for recurrent Clostridium difficile colitis, an underused treatment modality. Acta Gastroenterol Belg 2009;72:269–70.
28. MacConachie AA, Fox R, Kennedy DR, et al. Faecal transplant for recurrent Clostridium difficile-associated diarrhoea: a UK case series. QJM 2009;102: 781–4.
29. Arkkila PE, Uusitalo-Seppälä R, Lehtola L, et al. Fecal bacteriotherapy for recurrent *Clostridium difficile* infection. Gastroenterology 2010;138:S5.
30. Khoruts A, Dicksved J, Jansson JK, et al. Changes in the composition of the human fecal microbiome after bacteriotherapy for recurrent Clostridium difficile-associated diarrhea. J Clin Gastroenterol 2010;44:354–60.
31. Yoon SS, Brandt LJ. Treatment of refractory/recurrent *C. difficile*-associated disease by donated stool transplanted via colonoscopy: a case series of 12 patients. J Clin Gastroenterol 2010;44:562–6.
32. Rohlke F, SUrawicz CM, Stollman N. Fecal flora reconstitution for recurrent *Clostridium difficile* infection: results and methodology. J Clin Gastroenterol 2010;44: 567–70.
33. Silverman MS, Davis I, Pillai DR. Success of self-administered home fecal transplantation for chronic *Clostridium difficile* Infection. Clin Gastroenterol Hepatol 2010;5:471–3.
34. Garborg K, Waagsbø B, Stallemo A, et al. Results of faecal donor instillation therapy for recurrent *Clostridium difficile*-associated diarrhoea. Scand J Infect Dis 2010;42:857–61.
35. Russel G, Kaplan J, Ferraro MJ, et al. Fecal bacteriotherapy for relapsing *Clostridium difficile* infection in a child: a proposed treatment protocol. Pediatrics 2010;126:e239–42.
36. Kelly C, De Leon L. Successful treatment of recurrent Clostridium difficile infection with donor stool administered at colonoscopy: a case series [abstract 366]. Am J Gastroenterol 2010;105:S135.
37. Mellow M, Kanatzar A. Colonoscopic fecal bacteriotherapy in the treatment of recurrent *Clostridium difficile* infection [abstract]. Am J Gastroenterol 2010;105: S135.

38. Kassam Z, Hundal R, Marshall JK, et al. Fecal transplantation via retention enemas is effective for recurrent or refractory *Clostridium difficile*-associated diarrhea. Gastroenterology 2010;138:S207–8.

39. Kelly CR, de Leon L, Jasutkar N. Fecal microbiota transplantation for relapsing *Clostridium difficile* infection in 26 patients: methodology and results. J Clin Gastroenterol 2012;46(2):145–9.

40. Hamilton MJ, Weingarden AR, Sadowsky MJ, et al. Standardized frozen preparation for transplantation of fecal microbiota for recurrent *Clostridium difficile* infection. Am J Gastroenterol 2012;107(5):761–7.

41. Mattila E, Uusitalo-Seppälä R, Wuorela M, et al. Fecal transplantation, through colonoscopy, is effective therapy for recurrent *Clostridium difficile* infection. Gastroenterology 2012;142(3):490–6.

42. Brandt LJ, Aroniadis OC, Mellow M, et al. Long-term follow-up of colonoscopic fecal microbiota transplant for recurrent *Clostridium difficile* infection. Am J Gastroenterol 2012;107(7):1079–87.

43. Pepin J, Valiquette L, Alary ME, et al. *Clostridium difficile*-associated diarrhea in a region of Quebec from 1991 to 2003: a changing pattern of disease severity. CMAJ 2004;171:466–72.

44. Niagara System Faces Government Control. CBC news. Available at: http://www.cbc.ca/news/health/story/2011/08/15/c-difficile-niagara-supervisor.html.

45. Sailhamer EA, Carson K, Chang Y, et al. Fulminant *Clostridium difficile* colitis. Arch Surg 2009;144(5):433–9.

46. Pepin J. Improving the treatment of *Clostridium difficile*-associated disease: where should we start? Clin Infect Dis 2006;43:553–5.

47. McFarland LV, Elmer GW, Surawicz CM. Breaking the cycle: treatment strategies for 163 cases of recurrent *Clostridium difficile* disease. Am J Gastroenterol 2002;97:1769–75.

48. Bartlett JG. Narrative review: the new epidemic of *Clostridium difficile*-associated enteric disease. Ann Intern Med 2006;145(10):758–64.

49. Louie TJ, Miller MA, Mullane KM, et al. Fidaxomicin versus vancomycin for *Clostridium difficile* infection. N Engl J Med 2011;364(5):422–31.

50. Lagrotteria D, Holmes S, Smieja M, et al. Prospective, randomized inpatient study of oral metronidazole versus oral metronidazole and rifampin for treatment of primary episode of *Clostridium difficile*-associated diarrhea. Clin Infect Dis 2006;43(5):547–52.

51. Apisarnthanarak A, Mundy LM. Intracolonic vancomycin for adjunctive treatment of severe *clostridium difficile* colitis: indications and precautions. J Infect Dis Antimicrob Agents 2005;22:21–6.

52. McFarland LV. Alternative treatments for *Clostridium difficile* disease: what really works? J Med Microbiol 2005;54(2):101–11.

53. Tolevamer: a novel, non-antibiotic drug being investigated for the treatment of the most common cause of nosocomial diarrhea. Available at: www.genzyme.com/corp/./genz_pdf_tolevamer_nonconfidential.pdf.

54. Riley TV, Thean S, Hool G, et al. First Australian isolation of epidemic *Clostridium difficile* PCR ribotype 027. Med J Aust 2009;190(12):706–8.

55. Richards M, Knox J, Elliott B, et al. Severe infection with *Clostridium difficile* PCR ribotype 027 acquired in Melbourne, Australia. Med J Aust 2011;194(7): 369–71.

56. State hospitals fall prey to a different superbug. Available at: http://www.theage.com.au/victoria/state-hospitals-fall-prey-to-a-difficult-superbug-20120525-1zads.html.

57. Grehan MJ, Leis SM, Campbell J, et al. Durable alteration of the colonic microbiota by the administration of donor fecal flora. J Clin Gastroenterol 2010;44:551–61.
58. Brandt LJ, Borody TJ, Campbell J. Endoscopic fecal microbiota transplantation "first-line" treatment for severe *Clostridium difficile* Infection? J Clin Gastroenterol 2011;45(8):655–7.
59. Fujimura KE, Slusher NA, Cabana MD, et al. Role of the gut microbiota in defining human health. Expert Rev Anti Infect Ther 2010;8(4):435–54.
60. Qin J, Ruiqiang L, Raes J, et al. A human gut microbial gene catalogue established by metagenomic sequencing. Nature 2010;464:59–65.
61. Backhed F, Ley RE, Sonnenburg JL, et al. Host-bacterial mutualism in the human intestine. Science 2005;307(5717):1915–20.
62. Sekirov I, Russell SL, Antunes CM, et al. Gut microbiota in health and disease. Physiol Rev 2010;90(3):859–904.
63. Van Der Waaj D. Colonization resistance of the digestive tract: clinical consequences and implications. J Antimicrob Chemother 1982;10:263–70.
64. Barna JC, Williams DH. The structure and mode of action of glycopeptide antibiotics of the vancomycin group. Annu Rev Microbiol 1984;38:339–57.
65. Le Blay G, Lacroix C, Zihler A, et al. In vitro inhibition activity of nisin A, nisin Z, pediocin PA-1 and antibiotics against common intestinal bacteria. Lett Appl Microbiol 2007;45(3):252–7.
66. Martinez-Medina M, Aldeguer X, Gonzalez-Huix F, et al. Abnormal microbiota composition in the ileocolonic mucosa of Crohn's disease patients as revealed by polymerase chain reaction-denaturing gradient gel electrophoresis. Inflamm Bowel Dis 2006;12(12):1136–45.
67. Fava F, Danese S. Intestinal microbiota in inflammatory bowel disease: friend or foe? World J Gastroenterol 2011;17(5):557–66.
68. Sokol H, Pigneur B, Watterlot L, et al. *Faecalibacterium prausnitzii* is an anti-inflammatory commensal bacterium identified by gut microbiota analysis of Crohn's disease patients. Proc Natl Acad Sci U S A 2008;105(43):16731–6.
69. Lupp C, Robertson ML, Wickham ME, et al. Host-mediated inflammation disrupts the intestinal microbiota and promotes the overgrowth of Enterobacteriaceae. Cell Host Microbe 2007;2(3):204.
70. Barman M, Unold D, Shifley K, et al. Enteric salmonellosis disrupts the microbial ecology of the murine gastrointestinal tract. Infect Immun 2008;76(3):907–15.
71. Podolsky DK. Inflammatory bowel disease. N Engl J Med 2002;347:417–29.
72. Campbell J, Borody TJ, Leis S. The many faces of Crohn's Disease: latest concepts in etiology. Open J Intern Med 2012. [Epub ahead of print].
73. Borody TJ, George L, Andrews P, et al. Bowel-flora alteration: a potential cure for inflammatory bowel disease and irritable bowel syndrome? Med J Aust 1989; 150:604.
74. Moussata D, Goetz M, Gloeckner A, et al. Confocal laser endomicroscopy is a new imaging modality for recognition of intramucosal bacteria in inflammatory bowel disease in vivo. Gut 2011;60:26–33.
75. Andrews PJ, Barnes P, Borody TJ. Chronic constipation reversed by restoration of bowel flora. A case and a hypothesis. Eur J Gastroenterol Hepatol 1992;4: 245–7.
76. Turnbaugh PJ, Ley RE, Mahowald MA, et al. An obesity-associated gut microbiome with increased capacity for energy harvest. Nature 2006;444:1027–31.
77. Larsen N, Vogensen FK, Van Den Berg FW, et al. Gut microbiota in human adults with type 2 diabetes differs from non-diabetic adults. PLoS One 2010;5(2): e9085.

78. Parracho H, Bingham MO, Gibson GR, et al. Differences between the gut micro-flora of children with autism spectrum disorders and that of healthy children. J Med Microbiol 2005;54(10):987–91.

79. Gower-Rousseau C, Reumaux D, Bellard M, et al. Remission of myasthenia gravis after proctocolectomy in a patient with ulcerative colitis. Am J Gastroenterol 1993;88(7):1136–8.

80. Edwards CJ. Commensal gut bacteria and the etiopathogenesis of rheumatoid arthritis. J Rheumatol 2008;35:1477–9.

81. Armougom F, Henry M, Vialettes B, et al. Monitoring bacterial community of human gut microbiota reveals an increase in *Lactobacillus* in obese patients and methanogens in anorexic patients. PLoS One 2009;4(9):e7125.

82. Ley RE, Backhed F, Turnbaugh P, et al. Obesity alters gut microbial ecology. Proc Natl Acad Sci U S A 2005;102(31):11070–5.

83. Vrieze A, Holleman F, Serlie MJ, et al. Metabolic effects of transplanting gut microbiota from lean donors to subjects with metabolic syndrome. EASD 2010;A90.

84. Ueki A, Otsuka M. Life style risks of Parkinson's disease: association between decreased water intake and constipation. J Neurol 2004;251(7):18–23.

85. Abbott RD, Petrovich H, White LR, et al. Frequency of bowel movements and the future risk of Parkinson's disease. Neurology 2001;57:456–62.

86. Borody TJ, Torres M, Campbell J, et al. Treatment of severe constipation improves Parkinson's Disease (PD) symptoms. Am J Gastroenterol 2009;S999.

87. Braak H, Del Tredechi K, Rüb U, et al. Staging of brain pathology related to sporadic Parkinson's disease. Neurobiol Aging 2003;24:197–211.

88. Borody TJ, Rosen DM, Torres M, et al. Myoclonus dystonia- affected by GI microbiota. Am J Gastroenterol 2011;106:S352.

89. Mazmanian SK, Liu CH, Tzianabos AO, et al. An immunomodulatory molecule of symbiotic bacteria directs maturation of the host immune system. Cell 2005;122:107–18.

90. Finegold S, Molitoris D, Song Y, et al. Gastrointestinal microflora studies in late-onset autism. Clin Infect Dis 2002;35:S6–16.

91. Finegold S. State of the art; microbiology in health and disease. Intestinal bacterial flora in autism. Anaerobe 2011;17:367–8.

92. Goodwin MS, Goodwin TC, Cowen MA. Malabsorption and cerebral dysfunction: a multivariate and comparative study of autistic children. J Autism Child Schizophr 1971;1(1):48–62.

93. Horvath K, Perman JA. Autism and gastrointestinal symptoms. Curr Gastroenterol Rep 2002;4(3):251–8.

94. Valicenti-McDermott M, McVicar K, Rapin I, et al. Frequency of gastrointestinal symptoms in children with autism spectrum disorders and association with family history of autoimmune disease. J Dev Behav Pediatr 2006;27:S128–36.

95. Song Y, Liu C, Finegold SM. Real-time PCR quanititation of clostridia in feces of autistic children. Appl Environ Microbiol 2004;70(11):6459–65.

96. Sandler RH, Finegold SM, Bolte ER, et al. Short-term benefit from oral vancomycin treatment of regressive-onset autism. J Child Neurol 2000;15(7):429–35.

97. Ziomber A, Juszczak K, Kaszuba-Zwionska J, et al. Magnetically induced vagus nerve stimulation and feeding behaviour in rats. J Physiol Pharmacol 2009;60(3):71–7.

98. Bravo JA, Forsythe P, Chew MV. Ingestion of *Lactobacillus* strain regulates emotional behaviour and central GABA receptor expression in a mouse via the vagus nerve. Proc Natl Acad Sci U S A 2011;108(38):16050–5.

99. McLean PG, Bergonzelli GE, Collins SM, et al. Targeting the microbiota-gut-brain axis to modulate behaviour: which bacterial strain will translate best to humans? Proc Natl Acad Sci U S A 2012;109(4):E174.

100. Bolte ER. Autism and *clostridium tetani*. Med Hypothesis 1998;51(2):133–44.

101. Borody TJ. Bacteriotherapy for chronic fatigue syndrome: a long-term follow up study. Presented at the 1995 CFS National Consensus Conference.

102. FDA AABB donor history questionnaire documents. Available at: http://www.fda.gov/downloads/BiologicsBloodVaccines/BloodBloodProducts/ApprovedProducts/LicensedProductsBLAs/BloodDonorScreening/UCM213552.pdf.

103. Aas J, Gessert CE, Bakken JS. Recurrent *Clostridium difficile* colitis: case series involving 18 patients treated with donor stool administered via a nasogastric tube. Clin Infect Dis 2002;34(3):346–53.

Probiotics in the Management of Functional Bowel Disorders
Promise Fulfilled?

Eamonn M.M. Quigley, MD, FRCP, FRCPI*

KEYWORDS

- Irritable bowel syndrome • Constipation • Bloating • Functional bowel disorders
- Microbiota • Probiotics

KEY POINTS

- Recent research findings have revealed a potential role for the microbiota and the host immune response in irritable bowel syndrome.
- The primacy of a disturbed microbiota or an altered immune response in the pathogenesis of irritable bowel syndrome remains to be defined.
- Meta-analyses suggest that probiotics, as a therapeutic category, have a beneficial effect in irritable bowel syndrome.
- Studies of specific strains indicate that although some probiotics may ameliorate individual IBS symptoms, few have a global benefit.
- More appropriately powered studies of longer duration are required on the efficacy of probiotics in irritable bowel syndrome.

INTRODUCTION

The term *functional bowel disorder* refers to a group of conditions that feature a variety of gastrointestinal symptoms, such as abdominal pain or discomfort, diarrhea, constipation, bloating, and distension, for which there is no obvious organic cause. Being thus based on a process of exclusion rather than on a diagnostic biomarker, those entities included within this umbrella term are, by default, less circumscribed than more traditional diagnostic entities. Consequently, patient groups encompassed within this term are heterogeneous, and their symptoms are likely to represent the impact of various, as yet undefined, causes. The combination of population heterogeneity, undefined pathophysiology, and diagnostic imprecision is a recipe for therapeutic failure and, undoubtedly, accounts, in large part, for the challenges that

Department of Medicine, Alimentary Pharmabiotic Centre, University College Cork, Cork, Ireland
* Department of Medicine, Clinical Sciences Building, Cork University Hospital, Cork, Ireland.
E-mail address: e.quigley@ucc.ie

Gastroenterol Clin N Am 41 (2012) 805–819
http://dx.doi.org/10.1016/j.gtc.2012.08.005
0889-8553/12/$ – see front matter © 2012 Elsevier Inc. All rights reserved.

these disorders have presented to those who seek to develop new therapies. If therapy cannot be targeted on a well-characterized population whose problem is based on a disease process that is addressed by the new therapeutic entity, expectations for success must be low.

Some progress has been made, however, and concerted efforts to provide reproducible clinical definitions of subgroups within functional bowel disorders have produced more coherent populations. The most widely accepted and best validated of such approaches, the Rome process (now about to embark on its fourth iteration), has provided the clinical investigator with a classification of functional bowel disorders based on presenting symptoms: irritable bowel syndrome (IBS), functional (often referred to as *chronic*) constipation, functional diarrhea, and functional bloating.

Foremost is IBS, a common disorder worldwide[1] usually defined by the coexistence of abdominal pain or discomfort and an alteration in bowel habit.[2–4] IBS may lead to impaired social and personal function and can diminish quality of life to a degree usually associated with major organic diseases such as hypertension and diabetes.[1,5,6] IBS continues to represent a significant therapeutic challenge; currently available therapies provide symptomatic relief, at best, and none have been found to alter the natural history of the disorder.[2,3,7,8] According to Rome III, IBS is subtyped based on predominant bowel habit as diarrhea predominant, constipation predominant (IBS-C) and mixed type (formerly referred to as alternating IBS).[4]

Functional constipation represents the other well-characterized (and studied) functional disorder. Like IBS, its definition requires that symptoms (straining, lumpy or hard stools, sensation of incomplete evacuation, sensation of anorectal obstruction/blockage, use of manual maneuvers to facilitate defecation or infrequent defecation [<3 defecations/wk]) be present at a certain frequency (more than 25% of the time) and for a minimum length of time (3 months) with symptom onset at least 6 months earlier.[4] At times, the separation of functional (or chronic) constipation (CC) from IBS-C may pose a challenge, and debate continues as to whether these are overlapping disorders or part of a continuum. The prominence of pain in IBS traditionally is used as a differentiating factor; assigning the appropriate category to the patient with constipation, abdominal discomfort, and bloating is more challenging.

Drug discovery pathways and clinical trialists tend to treat these entities, IBS-C and CC, separately; accordingly, they will be addressed separately in this article. Because there have been few studies of probiotics in the other functional disorders (eg, functional bloating), these are discussed *en passant* in the context of IBS.

A SCIENTIFIC BASIS FOR THE USE OF PROBIOTICS IN FUNCTIONAL BOWEL DISORDERS
Irritable Bowel Syndrome

The precise pathophysiology of IBS remains to be elucidated.[9] For some time, pathophysiologic and pharmacologic research efforts focused on 2 principal targets: dysmotility[10,11] and altered visceral sensation.[12] Although there is no doubt that IBS is associated with several disturbances in motor function, not only in the colon, but throughout the gastrointestinal tract, and that visceral hypersensitivity is a common phenomenon in IBS, it seems unlikely that they represent fundamental pathophysiologic mechanisms.[13]

More recently, roles for enteric infection and intestinal inflammation have been proposed. Thus, both retrospective and prospective studies have documented the new onset of IBS after bacteriologically confirmed bacterial gastroenteritis[14,15]; postinfectious irritable bowel syndrome (PI-IBS) is not a transient entity but may cause long-lasting symptoms.[16] Furthermore, several risk factors for the development of PI-IBS have been identified.[15,17] Although results have not always been consistent,[18–20] others have described low-grade mucosal inflammation and immune activation in IBS in general[21–32] as well as evidence of microbe-host engagement.[33,34]

The enteric flora has also been implicated in the pathogenesis of non–PI-IBS.[35] First came the suggestion that some patients with IBS may harbor bacterial overgrowth and that their symptoms may be ameliorated by its eradication.[36,37] However, this proposal has met with considerable skepticism, and several subsequent studies have failed to confirm the original findings.[38–43] More recently, the focus has shifted to the colonic microbiota, and several studies using high-throughput sequencing approaches have described differences in the microbiota in IBS.[44–47] These observations, coupled with our ever-increasing understanding of gut flora-mucosa interactions,[48] including in IBS,[35] and the existence of a significant body of basic research to support a role for inflammatory and immune processes in contributing to enteric neuromuscular dysfunction,[49] have resulted in microbiota-host interactions gaining considerable credibility in explaining the pathophysiology of IBS and the precipitation of its symptoms.

Why use probiotics in IBS?

Probiotics, defined as live or attenuated bacteria or bacterial products that confer a significant health benefit to the host,[50] have the potential to provide a clinical tool to explore interactions between the resident flora, the intestinal epithelium, and the gut- or mucosa-associated lymphoid tissue. There are several reasons why these agents might, in theory, prove therapeutically beneficial in IBS.

Antibacterial and antiviral effects Many probiotic organisms exert antibacterial and antiviral effects and could, thereby, prevent or modify the course of postinfective IBS. Probiotics have been found to be beneficial in the prevention of human diarrheal conditions, such as toddlers' diarrhea[51] and antibiotic-associated diarrhea, including that related to *Clostridium difficile*.[52] These effects could be especially relevant to post-infectious IBS. Although probiotics have not been evaluated in the context of postinfectious IBS, the ability of probiotic preparations to influence the outcome of bacterial infections, such as *C difficile* colitis, and viral infections, such as rotavirus diarrhea, and the experimental demonstration of bacteriocidal, toxin-neutralizing, and antiviral effects for specific probiotic strains, suggest that probiotics may have a role in the prevention or treatment of postinfectious IBS.

Anti-inflammatory effects IBS may also be associated with inflammation or immune activation in the absence of an infectious trigger. That inflammation could lead to altered enteric nerve or muscle function had been amply shown in the past in such disorders as Chagas' disease and postviral gastroparesis. Furthermore, IBS-type symptoms also have been associated with inflammatory bowel disease[53] and celiac disease,[54] even when in apparent remission. Coupled with the aforementioned data to suggest activation of mast cells and lymphocytes in the colonic mucosa and elevated proinflammatory cytokine levels in the systemic circulation, a plausible hypothesis has emerged to suggest a role for immune dysfunction or low-grade inflammation in IBS.[22] Caution must be exercised, however, as results regarding mast cell and lymphocyte numbers have been variable[18]; immune dysfunction associated with a disrupted intestinal barrier may be more universally relevant to IBS.[18,19,55–58] Alterations in systemic cytokines also have not been documented consistently,[20,28–30] and the impact of central factors, such as stress,[32] must also be borne in mind before attributing a causal role to cytokines.

Laboratory experiments have repeatedly found the anti-inflammatory effects of certain probiotics. For example, oral administration of a *Bifidobacterium* exerted a profound anti-inflammatory effect in the interleukin (IL)-10 knock-out mouse, a potent model of inflammatory bowel disease that was associated with a suppression of the proinflammatory cytokines interferon-γ, tumor necrosis factor-α, and IL-12, while preserving activity of the anti-inflammatory cytokine transforming growth factor-β.[59,60] Others have found similar effects for the probiotic cocktail VSL#3 in another animal model of colitis; in this instance, the anti-inflammatory effect was evident with bacterial DNA alone.[61] In clinical practice, probiotics have been found to prevent the development of pouchitis[62] and reduce the relapse rate of this condition after successful antibiotic treatment.[63,64] By reducing mucosal inflammation, probiotics could decrease immune-mediated activation of enteric motor and sensory neurons and modify neural traffic between the gut and the central nervous system. There is some preliminary evidence that specific probiotics can diminish visceral hypersensitivity in animal models,[65,66] whereas others can reverse changes in intestinal muscle function induced by inflammation consequent on infection of an animal model with *Trichinella spiralis*.[67] Furthermore, several probiotics have been found to restore intestinal barrier function in various animal models.[68–71]

Evidence of immunologic effects in vivo in humans is limited; the most complete data coming from studies on *Bifidobacterium infantis* 35624, which found not only that this probiotic engaged with dendritic cells but that its consumption led to an augmentation of levels of the anti-inflammatory cytokine IL-10 in the systemic circulation in healthy volunteers,[72] indicating that this particular strain is capable of exerting immunoregulatory effects in man.[73] These findings are of particular relevance to IBS because this same probiotic has been found to ameliorate IBS symptoms in 2 randomized, controlled clinical trials.[28,74]

Altering the composition of the gut flora, effects on luminal contents Changes in the composition of the microbiota as a consequence of the administration of probiotics could, given the various and important metabolic functions of the microbiota, such as fermentation,[75] bile salt deconjugation,[76] and mucus degradation,[77] alter the volume or composition of colonic gas, influence stool consistency, or increase intestinal mucus secretion; effects that could influence intestinal handling of its contents and thus modulate such symptoms as constipation and diarrhea.

Effects on gut flora and luminal contents are not mutually exclusive and could also interact with other factors, such as diet, which are known to influence symptom onset in IBS. There is great interest in the role of diet and such dietary constituents as FODMAPS (fermentable, oligo-, di-, mono-saccharides and polyols)[78] and gluten[79] in the genesis of IBS symptomatology. Qualitative changes in the gut flora with a shift toward more gas-producing organisms, could interact with unabsorbed carbohydrates (such as in the patient with lactase deficiency or fructose intolerance) to increase colonic fermentation, which could not only increase intestinal gas-related symptoms, but also affect function in the proximal gut by promoting gastroesophageal reflux[80] and modifying proximal gastric relaxation.[81] These latter effects could contribute to the well-recognized overlap between IBS and other functional gastrointestinal disorders, such as nonerosive gastroesophageal reflux disease and functional dyspepsia.

Modulation of the gut-brain axis The concept of the brain-gut axis has been applied widely to IBS, and a variety of experimental and clinical observations have supported the importance of bidirectional interactions between the gut and the brain in the pathophysiology of IBS and the accentuation of its symptoms[82]; more novel has been the recent suggestion that this model could be extended to incorporate the microbiota: the microbiota-gut-brain axis.[83,84] Although considerable experimental evidence has been advanced to support this model,[85–88] its clinical relevance has yet to be defined.

Functional (Chronic) Constipation

The pathophysiology of CC is equally complex and undoubtedly encompasses at least 2 often overlapping entities: slow transit constipation and difficult defecation (also referred to as *anismus*). The former is assumed to be based primarily on colonic hypo-motility, the latter, on a disturbance in the coordination of the various entities that normally promote a successful act of defecation: the anatomic arrangement of the ano-rectum, the anal sphincters, the pelvic floor musculature, the abdominal muscles and the diaphragm. Although it is evident that symptoms are far-from-perfect predictors of underlying pathophysiology and that these 2 entities commonly coexist, therapeutic strategies have, traditionally, attempted to address one or the other, for example, prokinetics for slow transit constipation and biofeedback for anismus.

Why use probiotics in CC?

Given the impact of fiber and fiber supplements on the colonic microbiota and that the use of prebiotics and probiotics is presumed to be based on their ability to modify this population of microorganisms, one would assume that the role of microbiota-host interactions in a disorder as common as constipation is well defined; however, little is known of either quantitative or qualitative changes in bacteria or other organisms in this condition.

Zoppi and colleagues[89] reported increased numbers of clostridia and bifidobacteria among children with constipation, whereas Khalif and colleagues[90] noted that populations of lactobacilli and bifidobacteria were reduced among their adult subjects. Zoppi and colleagues,[89] while noting a modest symptomatic improvement with the administration of calcium polycarbophil, failed to detect an impact of this fiber analogue on the colonic microbiota. In a more indirect piece of evidence, Celik and colleagues[91] found that a course of vancomycin to constipated patients increased stool volume, frequency, consistency, and ease of defecation.

Recently, an impact of the small intestinal microbiota on constipation has been suggested by studies reporting that the excretion of abnormal amounts of methane after the administration of lactulose as part of a lactulose breath test to detect small intestinal bacterial overgrowth (SIBO) among subjects with IBS is associated with symptoms dominated by constipation (C-IBS). Although the status of SIBO in IBS remains a controversial issue, the association between methane excretion and constipation in IBS has been reasonably consistent.[36,37,41,92–94] In the study by Attaluri and colleagues,[94] methane production was more prevalent and higher among slow-transit than normal-transit constipation, again, supporting the idea that methane can slow gut transit.[93] It must be stressed that the origin of methane (or for that matter hydrogen) that is excreted in expired air in excess among these and other study subjects with constipation and C-IBS remains to be defined, and some would contend that this signal originates from colonic and not small intestinal methanogens.

These observations notwithstanding, the database on the microbiota and host-microbiota in chronic constipation, apart from the constipated variety of IBS, remains scanty.[57] That modulation of the microbiota might benefit constipated individuals and those with slow-transit constipation, in particular, is suggested by studies in animal models[95,96] and humans, which indicate the ability of certain probiotic strains to stimulate motility and peristalsis[95,96] and accelerate gut transit.[97–100]

CLINICAL STUDIES OF PROBIOTICS IN FUNCTIONAL BOWEL DISORDERS
Irritable Bowel Syndrome

Up to the year 2000, a small number of studies evaluated the response of IBS to probiotic preparations and, although results between studies were difficult to compare because of differences in study design, probiotic dose, and strain, there was some evidence of symptom improvement.[101] Most studies up to then were small in size and almost certainly underpowered to demonstrate anything other than a striking benefit. Several did not verify bacterial transit and survival by confirmatory stool studies. Many different organisms and strains were used, and dosages varied from as little as 10^5 to as many as 10^{13} colony forming units. Furthermore, some used probiotic cocktails rather than single isolates, rendering it difficult to induce what was/were the active moiety/moieties.

Further studies have assessed the response to several well-characterized organisms and have produced discernible trends. Thus, several organisms, such as *Lactobacillus GG, Lactobacillus plantarum, Lactobacillus acidophilus, Lactobacillus casei,* the probiotic cocktail VSL#3, and *Bifidobacterium animalis/lactis*, have been found to alleviate individual IBS symptoms, such as bloating, flatulence. and constipation.[28,73,99,102–110] Only a few products have been found to affect pain and global symptoms in IBS.[110–117] Results of other studies have been negative.[118,119]

Among the various species studied, *Bifidobacteria* have attracted particular attention.[117] Thus, *B infantis* 35624 was found to be superior to both a *Lactobacillus* and placebo for each of the cardinal symptoms of IBS (abdominal pain/discomfort, distension/bloating, and difficult defecation) and for a composite score.[28] A larger, 4-week, dose-ranging study of the same *Bifidobacterium* in more than 360 community-based subjects with IBS confirmed efficacy for this organism in a dose of 10^8; again, all of the primary symptoms of IBS were significantly improved, and a global assessment of IBS symptoms at the end of therapy found a greater than 20% therapeutic gain for the effective dose of the probiotic over placebo.[74] Another strain, *B lactis* DN-173-010A, has shown particular promise among IBS subjects with predominant constipation and prominent bloating[100,120]; the clinical effects of this strain on constipation and bloating have been supported by evidence that this bacterium accelerates colon transit and reduces abdominal distension.[100] Yet another bifidobacterial strain, *Bifidobacterium bifidum* MIMBb75, also proved effective in both symptom relief and improvement in quality of life.[121]

IBS typically is a chronic, relapsing condition, yet most studies of probiotics in this disorder have lasted no more than 408 weeks. Two longer-term studies (of 5 and 6 months' duration) involving the same probiotic cocktail did show a sustained, albeit modest, response.[122,123]

Further large, long-term, randomized, controlled trials of this *Bifidobacterium* and other strains are warranted in IBS, and detailed explorations of their mechanism(s) of action are indicated.

Chronic Constipation

Very few double-blind, placebo-controlled trials of probiotics in acute or chronic constipation (ie, other that in association with irritable bowel syndrome) are available. Among the few positive randomized, controlled trials are those of Koebnick and colleagues,[124] which documented a positive benefit for a probiotic beverage containing *L casei* Shirota, and of Yang and colleagues,[125] which reported benefits from *B.lactis* DN-173010, in patients with chronic constipation. In their study using *Lactobacillus* GG as an adjunct to lactulose, Banaszkiewicz and Szajewska[126] found no additional benefit from the probiotic. Coccorullo and colleagues[127] fed *Lactobacillus reuteri* (DSM 17938) or placebo to 44 consecutive infants who had a diagnosis of func-tional constipation and described a significant increase in stool frequency, although not in other constipation-related symptoms. Other studies, which were uncontrolled, or in which the probiotic was combined with some other form of therapy, reported vari-able benefits for bifidobacteria, lactobacilli, and *Propionibacteria* and infusions of fecal suspensions.[77,128–134] In a systematic review of probiotics in constipation, Chmielew-ska and Szajewska[135] identified only 5 randomized, controlled trials involving only 377 subjects.[135] The available data suggested a favorable effect of treatment with *B lactis* DN-173 010, *L casei* Shirota, and *Escherichia coli* Nissle 1917 on defecation frequency and stool consistency in adults. In children, *L casei* rhamnosus Lcr35, but not *Lacto-bacillus rhamnosus* GG, showed a beneficial effect. They concluded, however, that pending the arrival of more data, the use of probiotics for the treatment of constipation should be considered investigational.[135] Other, more recent reports have described benefits for probiotics in a variety of formulations[136–139]; comparisons among these studies are hampered by differences in study population, outcome measures, and probiotic strain, dose, and formulation.

THE FUTURE

The clear delineation of a postinfective variety of IBS and the evidence of low-grade inflammation and immune activation in IBS suggest a role for a dysfunctional relation-ship between the indigenous flora and the host in IBS and, accordingly, provide a clear rationale for the use of probiotics in this disorder. Other modes of action, including bacterial displacement and alterations in luminal contents, are also plausible. Clinical evidence of efficacy remains patchy, and although high-quality trials are now emerging, more long-term studies, which clearly define optimal strain, dose, and formulation, are needed. Probiotics, in general, seem to be most effective for symp-toms of bloating and flatulence, and certain strains seem to have more global effects; because of their good safety record, some authorities are now including probiotics in their dietary recommendations for the management of IBS.[140] The role of the micro-biota in chronic constipation is poorly understood, and data on the use of probiotics for this indication remain scanty.

ACKNOWLEDGMENTS

Supported, in part, by a grant from Science Foundation Ireland to the Alimentary Pharmabiotic Center.

REFERENCES

1. Quigley EM, Abdel-Hamid H, Barbara G, et al. A global perspective on irritable bowel syndrome: a consensus statement of the world gastroenterology organi-sation summit task force on irritable bowel syndrome. J Clin Gastroenterol 2012; 46:356–66.
2. Brandt LJ, Locke GR, Olden K, et al. An evidence-based approach to the management of irritable bowel syndrome in North America. Am J Gastroenterol 2002;97(Suppl):S1–26.
3. Drossman DA, Camilleri M, Mayer EA, et al. AGA technical review on irritable bowel syndrome. Gastroenterology 2002;123:2108–31.
4. Longstreth GF, Thompson WG, Chey WD, et al. Functional bowel disorders. Gastroenterology 2006;130:1480–91.

5. Thompson WG, Heaton KW, Smyth GT, et al. Irritable bowel syndrome in general practice: prevalence, characteristics, and referral. Gut 2000;46:78–82.

6. Hungin AP, Whorwell PJ, Tack J, et al. The prevalence, patterns and impact of irritable bowel syndrome: an international survey of 40,000 subjects. Aliment Pharmacol Ther 2003;17:643–50.

7. Brandt LJ, Chey WD, Foxx-Orenstein AE, et al, American College of Gastroenterology Task Force on Irritable Bowel Syndrome. An evidence-based position statement on the management of irritable bowel syndrome. Am J Gastroenterol 2009;104(Suppl 1):S1–35.

8. Ruepert L, Quartero AO, de Wit NJ, et al. Bulking agents, antispasmodics and antidepressants for the treatment of irritable bowel syndrome. Cochrane Database Syst Rev 2011;(8):CD003460.

9. Quigley EM. Current concepts of the irritable bowel syndrome. Scand J Gastroenterol 2003;38(Suppl 237):1–8.

10. McKee DP, Quigley EM. Intestinal motility and the irritable bowel syndrome - Is IBS a motility disorder? Part 1. Definition of IBS and colonic motility. Dig Dis Sci 1993;38:1761–72.

11. McKee DP, Quigley EM. Intestinal motility and the irritable bowel syndrome—is IBS a motility disorder? Part 2. Motility of the small bowel, esophagus, stomach and gall bladder. Dig Dis Sci 1993;38:1773–82.

12. Zhou Q, Verne GN. New insights into visceral hypersensitivity–clinical implications in IBS. Nat Rev Gastroenterol Hepatol 2011;8:349–55.

13. Quigley EM. Disturbances of motility and visceral hypersensitivity in irritable bowel syndrome: biological markers or epiphenomenon? Gastroenterol Clin North Am 2005;34:221–33.

14. Spiller R, Garsed K. Postinfectious irritable bowel syndrome. Gastroenterology 2009;136:1979–88.

15. Thabane M, Marshall JK. Post-infectious irritable bowel syndrome. World J Gastroenterol 2009;15:3591–6.

16. Marshall JK, Thabane M, Garg AX, et al. Walkerton Health Study Investigators. Eight year prognosis of postinfectious irritable bowel syndrome following waterborne bacterial dysentery. Gut 2010;59:605–11.

17. Villani AC, Lemire M, Thabane M, et al. Genetic risk factors for post-infectious irritable bowel syndrome following a waterborne outbreak of gastroenteritis. Gastroenterology 2010;138:1502–13.

18. Braak B, Klooker TK, Wouters MM, et al. Mucosal immune cell numbers and visceral sensitivity in patients with irritable bowel syndrome: is there any relationship? Am J Gastroenterol 2012;107:715–26.

19. Martínez C, Vicario M, Ramos L, et al. The jejunum of diarrhea-predominant irritable bowel syndrome shows molecular alterations in the tight junction signaling pathway that are associated with mucosal pathobiology and clinical manifestations. Am J Gastroenterol 2012;107:736–46.

20. Chang L, Adeyemo M, Karagiannides I, et al. Serum and colonic mucosal immune markers in irritable bowel syndrome. Am J Gastroenterol 2012;107:262–72.

21. Collins SM. A case for an immunological basis for irritable bowel syndrome. Gastroenterology 2002;122:2078–80.

22. Ohman L, Simrén M. Pathogenesis of IBS: role of inflammation, immunity and neuroimmune interactions. Nat Rev Gastroenterol Hepatol 2010;7:163–73.

23. Barbara G, Stanghellini V, De Giorgio R, et al. Activated mast cells in proximity to colonic nerves correlate with abdominal pain in irritable bowel syndrome. Gastroenterology 2004;126:693–702.

24. Barbara G, Wang B, Stanghellini V, et al. Mast cell-dependent excitation of visceral-nociceptive sensory neurons in irritable bowel syndrome. Gastroenterology 2007;132:26–37.

25. Cenac N, Andrews CN, Holzhausen M, et al. Role for protease activity in visceral pain in irritable bowel syndrome. J Clin Invest 2007;117:636–47.

26. Guilarte M, Santos J, de Torres I, et al. Diarrhoea-predominant IBS patients show mast cell activation and hyperplasia in the jejunum. Gut 2007;56:203–9.

27. Quigley EM. Therapies aimed at the gut microbiota and inflammation: antibiotics, prebiotics, probiotics, synbiotics, anti-inflammatory therapies. Gastroenterol Clin North Am 2011;40:207–22.

28. O'Mahony L, McCarthy J, Kelly P, et al. A Randomized, placebo-controlled, double-blind comparison of the probiotic bacteria lactobacillus and *Bifidobacterium* in irritable bowel syndrome (IBS): symptom responses and relationship to cytokine profiles. Gastroenterology 2005;128:541–51.

29. Liebregts T, Adam B, Bredack C, et al. Immune activation in patients with irritable bowel syndrome. Gastroenterology 2007;132:913–20.

30. Dinan TG, Quigley EM, Ahmed SM, et al. Hypothalamic–pituitary–gut axis dysregulation in irritable bowel syndrome: plasma cytokines as a potential biomarker? Gastroenterology 2006;130:304–11.

31. Scully P, McKernan DP, Keohane J, et al. Plasma cytokine profiles in females with irritable bowel syndrome and extra-intestinal co-morbidity. Am J Gastroenterol 2010;105:2235–43.

32. O'Malley D, Quigley EM, Dinan TG, et al. Do interactions between stress and immune responses lead to symptom exacerbations in irritable bowel syndrome? Brain Behav Immun 2011;25:1333–41.

33. McKernan DP, Gaszner G, Quigley EM, et al. Altered peripheral toll-like receptor responses in the irritable bowel syndrome. Aliment Pharmacol Ther 2011;33: 1045–52.

34. Brint EK, MacSharry J, Fanning A, et al. Differential expression of toll-like receptors in patients with irritable bowel syndrome. Am J Gastroenterol 2011;106: 329–36.

35. Ghoshal UC, Shukla R, Ghoshal U, et al. The gut microbiota and irritable bowel syndrome: friend or foe? Int J Inflam 2012;2012:151085.

36. Pimentel M, Chow EJ, Lin HC. Eradication of small bowel bacterial overgrowth reduces symptoms of irritable bowel syndrome. Am J Gastroenterol 2000;95: 3503–6.

37. Pimentel M, Chow E, Lin H. Normalization of lactulose breath testing correlates with symptom improvement in irritable bowel syndrome: a double-blind, randomized, placebo-controlled study. Am J Gastroenterol 2003;98:412–9.

38. Posserud I, Stotzer PO, Bjornsson E, et al. Small intestinal bacterial overgrowth in patients with irritable bowel syndrome. Gut 2006;56:802–8.

39. Vanner S. The small intestinal bacterial overgrowth. Irritable bowel syndrome hypothesis: implications for treatment. Gut 2008;57:1315–21.

40. Vanner S. The lactulose breath test for diagnosing SIBO in IBS patients: another nail in the coffin. Am J Gastroenterol 2008;103:964–5.

41. Bratten JR, Spanier J, Jones MP. Lactulose breath testing does not discriminate patients with irritable bowel syndrome from healthy controls. Am J Gastroenterol 2008;103:958–63.

42. Ford AC, Spiegel BM, Talley NJ, et al. Small intestinal bacterial overgrowth in irritable bowel syndrome: systematic review and meta-analysis. Clin Gastroenterol Hepatol 2009;7(12):1279–86.

43. Spiegel BM. Questioning the bacterial overgrowth hypothesis of irritable bowel syndrome: an epidemiologic and evolutionary perspective. Clin Gastroenterol Hepatol 2011;9:461–9.

44. Malinen E, Rinttilä T, Kajander K, et al. Analysis of the fecal microbiota of irritable bowel syndrome patients and healthy controls with real-time PCR. Am J Gastroenterol 2005;100:373–82.

45. Codling C, O'Mahony L, Shanahan F, et al. A molecular analysis of fecal and mucosal bacterial communities in irritable bowel syndrome. Dig Dis Sci 2010; 55:392–7.

46. Rajilić–Stojanović M, Biagi E, Heilig HG, et al. Global and deep molecular analysis of microbiota signatures in fecal samples from patients with irritable bowel syndrome. Gastroenterology 2011;141:1792–801.

47. Saulnier DM, Riehle K, Mistretta TA, et al. Gastrointestinal microbiome signatures of pediatric patients with irritable bowel syndrome. Gastroenterology 2011;141:1782–91.

48. Shanahan F. Therapeutic manipulation in gut flora. Science 2000;289:1311–2.

49. Collins SM. The immunomodulation of enteric neuromuscular function: implications for motility and inflammatory disorders. Gastroenterology 1996;111:1683–99.

50. Gorbach SL. Probiotics in the third millennium. Dig Liver Dis 2002;34(Suppl 2): S2–7.

51. Preidis GA, Hill C, Guerrant RL, et al. Probiotics, enteric and diarrheal diseases, and global health. Gastroenterology 2011;140:8–14.

52. Hempel S, Newberry SJ, Maher AR, et al. Probiotics for the prevention and treatment of antibiotic-associated diarrhea: a systematic review and meta-analysis. JAMA 2012;307:1959–69.

53. Keohane J, O'Mahony C, O'Mahony L, et al. Irritable bowel syndrome-type symptoms in patients with inflammatory bowel disease: a real association or reflection of occult inflammation? Am J Gastroenterol 2010;105:1788–94.

54. O'Leary C, Wieneke P, Buckley S, et al. Celiac disease and irritable bowel-type symptoms. Am J Gastroenterol 2002;97:1463–7.

55. Clarke G, Cryan JF, Dinan TG, et al. Review article: probiotics for the treatment of irritable bowel syndrome–focus on lactic acid bacteria. Aliment Pharmacol Ther 2012;35:403–13.

56. Quigley EM. Microflora modulation of motility. J Neurogastroenterol Motil 2011; 17:140–7.

57. Quigley EM. The enteric microbiota in the pathogenesis and management of constipation. Best Pract Res Clin Gastroenterol 2011;25:119–26.

58. Theoharides TC, Asadi S, Chen J, et al. Editorial: irritable bowel syndrome and the elusive mast cells. Am J Gastroenterol 2012;107:727–9.

59. O'Mahony L, Feeney M, O'Halloran S, et al. Probiotic impact on microbial flora, inflammation, and tumour development in IL-10 knockout mice. Aliment Pharmacol Ther 2001;15:1219–25.

60. McCarthy J, O'Mahony L, O'Callaghan L, et al. Double blind, placebo controlled trial of two probiotic strains in interleukin 10 knockout mice and mechanistic link with cytokine balance. Gut 2003;52:975–80.

61. Rachmilewitz D, Katakura K, Karmeli F, et al. Toll-like receptor 9 signaling mediates the anti-inflammatory effects of probiotics in murine experimental colitis. Gastroenterology 2004;126:520–8.

62. Gionchetti P, Rizzello F, Helwig U, et al. Prophylaxis of pouchitis onset with probiotic therapy: a double-blind, placebo-controlled trial. Gastroenterology 2003; 124:1202–9.

63. Gionchetti P, Rizzello F, Venturi A, et al. Oral bacteriotherapy as maintenance treatment in patients with chronic pouchitis: a double-blind, placebo-controlled trial. Gastroenterology 2000;119:305–9.

64. Mimura T, Rizzello F, Helwig U, et al. Once daily high dose probiotic therapy (VSL#3) for maintaining remission in recurrent or refractory pouchitis. Gut 2004;53:108–14.

65. Johnson AC, Greenwood-Van Meerveld B, McRorie J. Effects of *Bifidobacterium infantis* 35624 on post-inflammatory visceral hypersensitivity in the rat. Dig Dis Sci 2011;56:3179–86.

66. McKernan DP, Fitzgerald P, Dinan TG, et al. The probiotic *Bifidobacterium infantis* 35624 displays visceral antinociceptive effects in the rat. Neurogastroenterol Motil 2010;22:1029–35.

67. Verdu EF, Bercik P, Bergonzelli GE, et al. *Lactobacillus paracasei* normalizes muscle hypercontractility in a murine model of postinfective gut dysfunction. Gastroenterology 2004;127:826–37.

68. Jijon H, Backer J, Diaz H, et al. DNA from probiotic bacteria modulates murine and human epithelial and immune function. Gastroenterology 2004;126:1358–73.

69. Ait-Belgnaoui A, Han W, Lamine F, et al. *Lactobacillus farciminis* treatment suppresses stress induced visceral hypersensitivity: a possible action through interaction with epithelial cell cytoskeleton contraction. Gut 2006;55:1090–4.

70. Eutamene H, Lamine F, Chabo C, et al. Synergy between *Lactobacillus paracasei* and its bacterial products to counteract stress-induced gut permeability and sensitivity increase in rats. J Nutr 2007;137:1901–7.

71. Dai C, Guandalini S, Zhao DH, et al. Antinociceptive effect of VSL#3 on visceral hypersensitivity in a rat model of irritable bowel syndrome: a possible action through nitric oxide pathway and enhance barrier function. Mol Cell Biochem 2012;362:43–53.

72. Konieczna P, Groeger D, Ziegler M, et al. *Bifidobacterium infantis* 35624 administration induces Foxp3 T regulatory cells in human peripheral blood: potential role for myeloid and plasmacytoid dendritic cells. Gut 2012;61:354–66.

73. Konieczna P, Akdis CA, Quigley EM, et al. Portrait of an immunoregulatory Bifidobacterium. Gut Microbes 2012;3(3):261–6.

74. Whorwell PJ, Altringer L, Morel J, et al. Efficacy of an encapsulated probiotic *Bifidobacterium infantis* 35624 in women with irritable bowel syndrome. Am J Gastroenterol 2006;101:326–33.

75. Jiang T, Cavaiano DA. Modification of colonic fermentation by bifidobacteria and pH in vitro: impact on lactose metabolism, short-chain fatty acid, and lactate production. Dig Dis Sci 1997;42:2370–7.

76. Begley M, Hill C, Gahan CG. Bile salt hydrolase activity in probiotics. Appl Environ Microbiol 2006;72:1729–38.

77. Ouwehand AC, Lagstrom H, Suomalainen T, et al. Effect of probiotics on constipation, fecal azoreductase activity and fecal mucin content in the elderly. Ann Nutr Metab 2002;46:159–62.

78. Ong DK, Mitchell SB, Barrett JS, et al. Manipulation of dietary short chain carbohydrates alters the pattern of gas production and genesis of symptoms in irritable bowel syndrome. J Gastroenterol Hepatol 2010;25:1366–73.

79. Biesiekierski JR, Newnham ED, Irving PM, et al. Gluten causes gastrointestinal symptoms in subjects without celiac disease: a double-blind randomized placebo-controlled trial. Am J Gastroenterol 2011;106:508–14.

80. Piche T, des Varannes SB, Sacher-Huvelin S, et al. Colonic fermentation influences lower esophageal sphincter function in gastroesophageal reflux disease. Gastroenterology 2003;124:894–902.
81. Ropert A, Cherbut C, Roze C, et al. Colonic fermentation and proximal gastric tone in humans. Gastroenterology 1996;111:289–96.
82. Camilleri M, Di Lorenzo C. Brain-gut axis: from basic understanding to treatment of IBS and related disorders. J Pediatr Gastroenterol Nutr 2012;54:446–53.
83. Cryan JF, O'Mahony SM. The microbiome-gut-brain axis: from bowel to behavior. Neurogastroenterol Motil 2011;23:187–92.
84. Grenham S, Clarke G, Cryan JF, et al. Brain-gut-microbe communication in health and disease. Front Physiol 2011;2:94.
85. Bravo JA, Forsythe P, Chew MV, et al. Ingestion of lactobacillus strain regulates emotional behavior and central GABA receptor expression in a mouse via the vagus nerve. Proc Natl Acad Sci U S A 2011;108:16050–5.
86. Bercik P, Park AJ, Sinclair D, et al. The anxiolytic effect of *Bifidobacterium longum* NCC3001 involves vagal pathways for gut-brain communication. Neurogastroenterol Motil 2011;23:1132–9.
87. Bercik P, Denou E, Collins J, et al. The intestinal microbiota affect central levels of brain-derived neurotropic factor and behavior in mice. Gastroenterology 2011;141:599–609.
88. Heijtz RD, Wang S, Anuar F, et al. Normal gut microbiota modulates brain development and behavior. Proc Natl Acad Sci U S A 2011;108:3047–52.
89. Zoppi G, Cinquetti M, Luciano A, et al. The intestinal ecosystem in chronic functional constipation. Acta Paediatr 1998;87:836–41.
90. Khalif IL, Konovitch EA, Maximova ID, et al. Alterations in the colonic flora and intestinal permeability and evidence of immune activation in chronic constipation. Dig Liver Dis 2005;37:838–49.
91. Celik AF, Tomlin J, Read NW. The effect of oral vancomycin on chronic idiopathic constipation. Aliment Pharmacol Ther 1995;9:63–8.
92. Hwang L, Low K, Khoshini R, et al. Evaluating breath methane as a diagnostic test for constipation-predominant IBS. Dig Dis Sci 2010;55:398–403.
93. Sahakian AB, Jee SR, Pimentel M. Methane and the gastrointestinal tract. Dig Dis Sci 2010;55:2135–43.
94. Attaluri A, Jackson M, Valestin J, et al. Methanogenic flora is associated with altered colonic transit but not stool characteristics in constipation without IBS. Am J Gastroenterol 2010;105:1407–11.
95. Lesniewska V, Rowland I, Laerke HN, et al. Relationship between dietary-induced changes in intestinal commensal microflora and duodenojejunal myoelectric activity monitored by radiotelemetry in the rat in vivo. Exp Physiol 2006;91:229–37.
96. Matsumoto M, Ishige A, Yazawa Y, et al. Promotion of intestinal peristalsis by *Bifidobacterium* spp. Capable of hydrolysing sennosides in mice. PLoS One 2012;7:e31700.
97. Marteau P, Cuillerier E, Meance S, et al. *Bifidobacterium animalis* strain DN-173 010 shortens the colonic transit time in healthy women: a double-blind, randomized, controlled study. Aliment Pharmacol Ther 2002;16:587–93.
98. Bouvier M, Meance S, Bouley C, et al. Effects of consumption of a milk fermented by the probiotic strain *Bifidobacterium animalis* DN-173 010 on colonic transit times in healthy humans. Biosci Microflora 2001;20:43–8.
99. Meance S, Cayuela C, Turchet P, et al. A fermented milk with a *Bifidobacterium* probiotic strain DN-173 010 shortened oro-fecal gut transit time in elderly. Microb Ecol Health Dis 2001;13:217–22.

100. Agrawal A, Houghton LA, Morris J, et al. Clinical trial: the effects of a fermented milk product containing *Bifidobacterium lactis* DN-173-010 on abdominal distension and gastrointestinal transit in irritable bowel syndrome with constipation. Aliment Pharmacol Ther 2009;29:104–14.
101. Hamilton-Miller JM. Probiotics in the management of irritable bowel syndrome: a review of clinical trials. Microb Ecol Health Dis 2001;13:212–6.
102. Nobaek S, Johansson ML, Molin G, et al. Alteration of intestinal microflora is associated with reduction in abdominal bloating and pain in patients with irritable bowel syndrome. Am J Gastroenterol 2000;95:1231–8.
103. O'Sullivan MA, O'Morain CA. Bacterial supplementation in the irritable bowel syndrome. A randomised double-blind placebo-controlled crossover study. Dig Liver Dis 2000;32:302–4.
104. Brigidi P, Vitali B, Swennen E, et al. Effects of probiotic administration upon the composition and enzymatic activity of human fecal microbiota in patients with irritable bowel syndrome or functional diarrhea. Res Microbiol 2001;152:735–41.
105. Niedzielin K, Kordecki H, Birkenfeld B. A controlled, double-blind, randomized study on the efficacy of *Lactobacillus plantarum* 299V in patients with irritable bowel syndrome. Eur J Gastroenterol Hepatol 2001;13:1143–7.
106. Sen S, Mullan MM, Parker TJ, et al. Effect of *Lactobacillus plantarum* 299v on colonic fermentation and symptoms of irritable bowel syndrome. Dig Dis Sci 2002;47:2615–20.
107. Bazzocchi G, Gionchetti P, Almerigi PF, et al. Intestinal microflora and oral bacteriotherapy in irritable bowel syndrome. Dig Liver Dis 2002;34(Suppl 2):s48–53.
108. Kim HJ, Camilleri M, McKinzie S, et al. A randomized controlled trial of a probiotic, VSL#3, on gut transit and symptoms in diarrhoea-predominant irritable bowel syndrome. Aliment Pharmacol Ther 2003;17:895–904.
109. Ringel-Kulka T, Palsson OS, Maier D, et al. Probiotic bacteria lactobacillus acidophilus NCFM and *Bifidobacterium lactis* Bi-07 versus placebo for the symptoms of bloating in patients with functional bowel disorders: a double-blind study. J Clin Gastroenterol 2011;45:518–25.
110. Horvath A, Dziechciarz P, Szajewska H. Meta-analysis: *Lactobacillus rhamnosus* GG for abdominal pain-related functional gastrointestinal disorders in childhood. Aliment Pharmacol Ther 2011;33:1302–10.
111. Ki Cha B, Mun Jung S, Hwan Choi C, et al. The effect of a multispecies probiotic mixture on the symptoms and fecal microbiota in diarrhea-dominant irritable bowel syndrome: a randomized, double-blind, placebo-controlled trial. J Clin Gastroenterol 2012;46:220–7.
112. Choi CH, Jo SY, Park HJ, et al. A randomized, double-blind, placebo-controlled multicenter trial of saccharomyces boulardii in irritable bowel syndrome: effect on quality of life. J Clin Gastroenterol 2011;45:679–83.
113. Nikfar S, Rahimi R, Rahimi F, et al. Efficacy of probiotics in irritable bowel syndrome: a meta-analysis of randomized, controlled trials. Dis Colon Rectum 2008;51:1775–80.
114. McFarland LV, Dublin S. Meta-analysis of probiotics for the treatment of irritable bowel syndrome. World J Gastroenterol 2008;14:2650–61.
115. Hoveyda N, Heneghan C, Mahtani KR, et al. A systematic review and meta-analysis: probiotics in the treatment of irritable bowel syndrome. BMC Gastroenterol 2009;9:15.
116. Moayyedi P, Ford AC, Talley NJ, et al. The efficacy of probiotics in the therapy of irritable bowel syndrome: a systematic review. Gut 2008;59(3):325–32.

117. Brenner DM, Moeller MJ, Chey WD, et al. The utility of probiotics in the treatment of irritable bowel syndrome: a systematic review. Am J Gastroenterol 2009; 104(4):1033–49 [quiz: 1050].

118. Kabir MA, Ishaque SM, Ali MS, et al. Role of saccharomyces boulardii in diarrhea predominant irritable bowel syndrome. Mymensingh Med J 2011;20: 397–401.

119. Søndergaard B, Olsson J, Ohlson K, et al. Effects of probiotic fermented milk on symptoms and intestinal flora in patients with irritable bowel syndrome: a randomized, placebo-controlled trial. Scand J Gastroenterol 2011;46:663–72.

120. Guyonnet D, Chassany O, Ducrotte P, et al. Effect of a fermented milk containing Bifidobacterium animalis DN-173 010 on the health-related quality of life and symptoms in irritable bowel syndrome in adults in primary care: a multicentre, randomized, double-blind, controlled trial. Aliment Pharmacol Ther 2007;26: 475–86.

121. Guglielmetti S, Mora D, Gschwender M, et al. Randomised clinical trial: Bifidobacterium bifidum MIMBb75 significantly alleviates irritable bowel syndrome and improves quality of life–a double-blind, placebo-controlled study. Aliment Pharmacol Ther 2011;33:1123–32.

122. Kajander K, Hatakka K, Poussa T, et al. A probiotic mixture alleviates symptoms in irritable bowel syndrome patients: a controlled 6-month intervention. Aliment Pharmacol Ther 2005;22:387–94.

123. Kajander K, Myllyluoma E, Rajilić-Stojanović M, et al. Clinical trial: multispecies probiotic supplementation alleviates the symptoms of irritable bowel syndrome and stabilizes intestinal microbiota. Aliment Pharmacol Ther 2008;27:48–57.

124. Koebnick C, Wagner I, Leitzmann P, et al. Probiotic beverage containing Lactobacillus casei shirota improves gastrointestinal symptoms in patients with chronic constipation. Can J Gastroenterol 2003;17:655–9.

125. Yang YX, He M, Hu G, et al. Effect of a fermented milk containing Bifidobacterium lactis DN-173010 on Chinese constipated women. World J Gastroenterol 2008;14:6237–43.

126. Banaszkiewicz A, Szajewska H. Ineffectiveness of Lactobacillus GG as an adjunct to lactulose for the treatment of constipation in children: a double-blind, placebo-controlled randomized trial. J Pediatr 2005;146:364–9.

127. Coccorullo P, Strisciuglio C, Martinelli M, et al. Lactobacillus reuteri (DSM 17938) in infants with functional chronic constipation: a double-blind, randomized, placebo-controlled study. J Pediatr 2010;157:598–602.

128. Amenta M, Cascio MT, Di Fiore P, et al. Diet and chronic constipation. Benefits of oral supplementation with symbiotic zir fos (Bifidobacterium longum W11 + FOS Actilight). Acta Biomed 2006;77:157–62.

129. De Paula JA, Carmuega E, Weill R. Effect of the ingestion of a symbiotic yogurt on the bowel habits of women with functional constipation. Acta Gastroenterol Latinoam 2008;38:16–25.

130. Bekkali NL, Bongers ME, Van den Berg MM, et al. The role of a probiotics mixture in the treatment of childhood constipation: a pilot study. Nutr J 2007;6:17.

131. Bu LN, Chang MH, Ni YH, et al. Lactobacillus casei rhamnosus Lcr35 in children with chronic constipation. Pediatr Int 2007;49:485–90.

132. Borody TJ, Warren EF, Leis SM, et al. Bacteriotherapy using fecal flora: toying with human motions. J Clin Gastroenterol 2004;38:475–83.

133. Pitkala KH, Strandberg TE, Finne Soveri UH, et al. Fermented cereal with specific bifidobacteria normalizes bowel movements in elderly nursing home residents. A randomized, controlled trial. J Nutr Health Aging 2007;11:305–11.

134. An HM, Baek EH, Jang S, et al. Efficacy of lactic acid bacteria (LAB) supplement in management of constipation among nursing home residents. Nutr J 2010;9:5.
135. Chmielewska A, Szajewska H. Systematic review of randomised controlled trials: probiotics for functional constipation. World J Gastroenterol 2010;16:69–75.
136. Guerra PV, Lima LN, Souza TC, et al. Pediatric functional constipation treatment with *Bifidobacterium*-containing yogurt: a crossover, double-blind, controlled trial. World J Gastroenterol 2011;17:3916–21.
137. Tabbers MM, Chmielewska A, Roseboom MG, et al. Fermented milk containing *Bifidobacterium lactis* DN-173 010 in childhood constipation: a randomized, double-blind, controlled trial. Pediatrics 2011;127:e1392–9.
138. Del Piano M, Carmagnola S, Anderloni A, et al. The use of probiotics in healthy volunteers with evacuation disorders and hard stools: a double-blind, randomized, placebo-controlled study. J Clin Gastroenterol 2010;44(Suppl 1):S30–4.
139. Riezzo G, Orlando A, D'Attoma B, et al. Randomised clinical trial: efficacy of *Lactobacillus paracasei*-enriched artichokes in the treatment of patients with functional constipation–a double-blind, controlled, crossover study. Aliment Pharmacol Ther 2012;35:441–50.
140. McKenzie YA, Alder A, Anderson W, et al, On behalf of Gastroenterology Specialist Group of the British Dietetic Association. British Dietetic Association evidence-based guidelines for the dietary management of irritable bowel syndrome in adults. J Hum Nutr Diet 2012;25:260–74.

Probiotic Bacteria in the Prevention and the Treatment of Inflammatory Bowel Disease

Richard Fedorak, MD, FRCP, FRCP(London), FRS*,
Denny Demeria, MD, FRCPC

KEYWORDS

- Inflammatory bowel disease • Crohn disease • Ulcerative colitis • Pouchitis
- Probiotics • Prebiotics • Synbiotics

KEY POINTS

- The gastrointestinal microbiota is highly diverse. Alterations in this microbiota have been show to both cause and abrogate systemic inflammatory disorders.
- Probiotics are defined as microbiotia that have a beneficial effect on human health.
- Recently, probiotics and probiotic preparations have been studied as therapeutic agents to modify the gastrointestinal microbiota and thereby treat inflammatory bowel diseases (IBDs).
- Randomized clinical trials have shown that select probiotics are efficacious for the induction and maintenance of remission in ulcerative colitis and for the maintenance of remission in pouchitis.
- Not all probiotics are the same or have similar efficacy. Adequately powered, randomized controlled clinical trials are required for each probiotic to confirm its efficacy in IBD.

INTRODUCTION

The traditional classification of IBD into Crohn disease and ulcerative colitis offers health care providers a logical and evidenced-based approach in developing a meaningful therapeutic approach for the prevention and treatment of these diseases. Current therapies may leave many patients and physicians frustrated, because persistent symptomatology and endoscopic or histopathologic evidence of active disease usually persist despite optimum medical and surgical management. As comprehension of these diseases has progressed, advanced pharmacologic biologic therapies have been developed, such as anti–tumor necrosis factor α (anti–TNF-α) agents,

---

The authors have nothing to disclose.
Division of Gastroenterology, University of Alberta, 2-14A Zeidler Building, 130 University Campus, Edmonton, Alberta T6G 2X8, Canada
* Corresponding author.
E-mail address: Richard.fedorak@ualberta.ca

Gastroenterol Clin N Am 41 (2012) 821–842
http://dx.doi.org/10.1016/j.gtc.2012.08.003
0889-8553/12/$ – see front matter © 2012 Elsevier Inc. All rights reserved.

which have resulted in improved symptom and disease control in many patients. Currently, however, a definitive curative strategy for these diseases, using medical therapy alone, remains elusive. Furthermore, these medications are not without significant cost nor are they without risk of potential, and often substantial, side effects. For these reasons, there is a prevalent interest in patients with IBD in pursuing nonconventional avenues of therapy for both symptoms and disease control.[1]

Given these considerations, there has been an increasing appreciation of the importance in understanding the complexities of the interactions between the human host immune system and its resident gastrointestinal luminal microbial population. Current models for the pathogenesis of IBD have demonstrated evidence for a disturbance in this equilibrium, resulting from either an aberrant host immune response to usual luminal microbiota,[2] an exaggerated physiologic immune phenomenon to an abnormal population of microbes in the gastrointestinal tract,[3] or a combination of both.

Probiotic organisms, which are defined as "live microorganisms which when administered in adequate amounts confer a health benefit on the host,"[4] have been used in attempts to take advantage of this relationship to treat various gastrointestinal diseases, including acute traveler's diarrhea,[5] infectious diarrhea,[6] and irritable bowel syndrome[7]; in the prevention of infantile necrotizing enterocolitis in neonates[8]; and to alter gut microflora in patients with minimal hepatic encephalopathy to prevent the growth of ammonia-producing bacteria in patients with hepatic cirrhosis.[9]

Although the spectrum of diseases of the intestines is broad, this article focuses on the actual and potential roles of the probiotic organism in patients with Crohn disease and ulcerative colitis. To begin with, the basic aspects of the enteric microorganism are reviewed, as they pertain to the development of IBD, and they are compared and contrasted with the host-specific responses to probiotic administration, in both the IBD and non-IBD host. Then the available clinical literature is reviewed, focusing on the use of probiotics in Crohn disease and ulcerative colitis, examining the roles of the probiotic organism in induction of remission as maintenance therapy and in the surgical patient with IBD. Finally, future roles of probiotic therapy in the realm of IBD are proposed.

GASTROINTESTINAL MICROBES AND IBD

The human gastrointestinal tract provides a suitable environment to a diverse microbial population, with more than 400 to 500 different species of bacteria currently identified.[10] The primary introduction of this array to the host most likely occurs in close relationship to labor and delivery of the neonate, with *Lactobacillus* and *Prevotella* spp predominating within the vaginal canal at the time of delivery.[11,12] Once established, this microbial population maybe susceptible to changes in diet,[13] age of the host,[14] disease states, and lifestyle. Nevertheless, the specific changes that are effected in the microbial population by each of these variables, however, remain to be fully elucidated.

The importance of the microbe in IBD is demonstrated by clinical and histologic improvement in fecal diversion in patients with Crohn disease[15]; recurrence of symptoms and inflammation with re-exposure of the terminal ileum to luminal contents is the rule. Several studies have magnified the importance of enteral microorganisms in the development and maintenance of IBD. Analysis of mucosal-associated and fecal bacteria reveals diminished commensal microbial diversity (decreased numbers of *Faecalibacterium prausnitzii* and *Lactobacillus*),[16–21] an increased number of mucosal-associated microorganisms,[22,23] and an orientation toward phylogenetic groups of proinflammatory microbes, such as *Escherichia coli,* in patients with active inflammation in Crohn disease and ulcerative colitis.[24,25] It remains to be seen whether this dysbiotic environment is a prerequisite for developing IBD or is a result of it and which bacteria are specifically involved.

To date, the identification of one or more causative organisms in IBD has not been found. Although early association of *Mycobacterium avium* subsp *paratuberculosis* with spontaneous granulomatous enterocolitis provided a potential causative organism for IBD,[26] its specific role in IBD remains to be determined.[27] Similarly, although there is a higher prevalence of *Yersinia* and *Camplyobacter* species in patients with Crohn disease compared with controls,[28,29] their roles too remain to be investigated. Particular attention has been paid to the presence of pathogenic adherent-invasive *E coli*, which has been identified in 36.4% of patients with Crohn disease versus 6% of controls.[30] The reasons for this difference most likely represent a combination of host characteristics (ie, Paneth cell dysfunction; genetic mutations in *NOD2, ATG16L1,* or *IRGM;* and abnormal ileal expression of carcinoembryonic antigen-related cell adhesion molecule 6) and microbial properties (type 1 pili variants and increased TNF-α and IFN-γ secretion). The specific relationships between the host immune system and microbiota in IBD are beyond the scope of this article and are reviewed elsewhere.[2,31]

The microbe and IBD recall points
- 400–500 Species of bacteria reside within human gastrointestinal tract.
- The human host is colonized at birth with bacteria from caregivers. The majority of the bacteria are constant whereas a small proportion can change with time and circumstance (age, disease, lifestyle, and so forth).
- IBD involves dysbiosis and/or abnormal immune host response to the dysbiosis.

PROBIOTICS

The alteration of the type or number of bacteria within the gastrointestinal tract in states of disease may have various effects on the host. Thus, the potential to manipulate enteric flora for positive therapeutic purposes is an attractive approach for patients with IBD. Probiotic organisms have had a history of both local and systemic beneficial effects.[32–34] **Box 1** summarizes the multiple beneficial effects, relative to IBD, which probiotic bacteria exert on the gastrointestinal tract. Examples of these were investigated in a pilot study,[35] which examined the effects of various *Lactobacilli* species on various mediators of inflammation and found that the intestinal *Lactobacilli* of elderly persons are tightly associated with increased serum white blood cell count (*Lactobacillus reuteri*), reduced blood glucose levels (*L fermentum*), and oxidized low-density lipoprotein content (various *Lactobacilli*). In another study, one specific probiotic mixture, VSL3, was found to enhance the anti-inflammatory cytokine pathway via induction of mucosal-associated CD425+ and CD4+ LAP cells[36] and reduce the level of proinflammatory cytokines, including TNF-α, interleukin 1β, and interferon γ.[37]

Not all probiotics have similar mechanisms of action and even those with proved efficacy in IBD may exhibit only a few of the beneficial mechanisms outlined in **Box 1**. Nevertheless, the ability of probiotics to modulate the microbial-intestinal–immune cascade, even on a minor scale, provides a rational basis for their use in patients with IBD.

Probiotics recall points
- Probiotics are microorganisms, which provide a benefit to the host.
- Probiotics have been shown to have both local and systemic effects on the host.
- Therapeutically successful probiotics have a predominantly anti-inflammatory effect.

Box 1
Biologic effects of probiotic bacteria

Host Immune Response Modulation	Epithelial Barrier Function Modulation	Antimicrobial Effects
• Enhanced antibody production and natural killer cell activity	• Enhanced tight junction protein phosphorylation	• Impeded bacterial adhesion to epithelial cell layer
• Modulation of dendritic cell phenotype	• Upregulation of mucus layer	• Upregulated defensin secretion
• Induction of peroxisome proliferator activated receptor-γ and T-regulatory cells	• Increased secretory immunoglobulin A production	• Antimicrobial peptide secretion
• Modulation of apoptosis	• Enhanced epithelial cell glycosylation	• Decreased intraluminal pH
• Inhibition of proteasome activity		• Inhibits pathogenic bacterial invasion
• Altered cytokine release		
• Modulation of nuclear factor κB and activator protein 1 pathways		

PROBIOTICS IN THE TREATMENT OF INFLAMMATORY BOWEL DISEASE
Ulcerative Colitis

Induction of remission

Currently, the data to support clear and consistent clinical benefits in inducing remission in patients with active ulcerative colitis are encouraging, although conflicting data exist (**Table 1**). The data for probiotics in the induction and maintenance of ulcerative colitis are summarized in **Table 1**.

Recently, Sood and colleagues[38] from India conducted a randomized, multicenter, double-blind, controlled trial evaluating twice-daily probiotic mixture, VSL3 (3.6×10^9 colony-forming units [CFU]), in inducing remission in 77 patients with mild to moderately severe ulcerative colitis versus 70 patients given placebo. The primary endpoint was a 50% decrease in ulcerative colitis disease activity index (UCDAI) score at 6 weeks, with final evaluation at 12 weeks. The percentage of patients achieving the primary endpoint was higher in the VSL3 group than the placebo group, both at week 6 (32.5% vs 10%, $P = .001$) and at week 12 (42.9% vs 15.7%, $P<.001$).

In a follow-up study, of similar design, Tursi and colleagues[39] sought to evaluate the utility of VSL3 in the treatment of relapsing-remitting mild to moderate ulcerative colitis in a double-blind, placebo-controlled trial involving 144 patients randomly treated for 8 weeks with VSL3 (3600 billion CFU/d) (71 patients) or with placebo (73 patients). As a secondary endpoint, 31 (47.7%) patients in the VLS3 group and 23 (32.4%) patients in the placebo group had remission induced by the end of 8 weeks, yet this difference did not reach statistical significance.

Given the potential efficacy of VSL3 in patients with ulcerative colitis, the authors examined its effect in 32 patients with active ulcerative colitis in 2005.[40] As an open-label trial, twice-daily dosing of 1800 billion bacteria was administered to patients, who were on concomitant medical therapy (steroids, 5-aminosalicylic acid

Table 1
Induction and maintenance of remission in ulcerative colitis: a summary of evidence investigating the effect of probiotic treatments

First Author, Year	Design Duration	Probiotic	Group (dose/d) Comparator	Concomitant Therapy	Results
Ulcerative colitis: induction of remission					
Rembacken et al,[42] 1999	DB, R, C 1 y	E coli Nissle 1917 (1×10^{11} CFU) n = 57	Mesalamine (2.4 g) n = 59	Prednisolone or hydrocortisone enemas	As effective as mesalamine at attaining remission
Borody et al,[81] 2003	Case reports 2–13 y	Fecal enema n = 6	None	None	100% Remission
Guslandi et al,[82] 2003	O 4 wk	S boulardii (750 mg) n = 25	None	Mesalamine	Reduction in UCDAI scores
Kato et al,[83] 2004	DB, R, C 12 wk	Bifidobacterium-fermented milk (100 mL) n = 10	Placebo n = 10	Sulfasalazine and mesalamine	Reduction in UCDAI ($P<.05$)
Tursi et al,[84] 2004	R, O 8 wk	Balsalazide (2.25 g) and VSL3 (1×10^{11} CFU) n = 30	Balsalazide (4.5 g) n = 30 Mesalamine (2.4 g) n = 28	None	Balsalazide and VSL3 outperformed the 2 comparator groups (symptoms assessment, endoscopic appearance, and histologic evaluation)
Bibiloni et al,[40] 2005	O 6 wk	VSL3 (3.6×10^9 CFU) n = 32	None	Mesalamine, steroids, or immunosuppressants	Remission (UCDAI $\leq$2) achieved in 18, response (UCDAI $\geq$3) achieved in 8 whereas 3 did not have a response and 3 others worsened
Furrie et al,[47] 2005	DB, R, C 1 mo	B longum and Synergy 1 n = 8	Placebo n = 8	Mesalamine, immunosuppressants, steroids	NSD re sigmoidoscopy scores

(continued on next page)

Table 1
(continued)

First Author, Year	Design Duration	Group (dose/d)		Concomitant Therapy	Results
		Probiotic	Comparator		
Tsuda et al,[41] 2007	O 4 wk	BIO-THREE n = 20	None	Mesalamine or 6-mercaptopurine	Remission achieved in 9/20 patients, no response in 8/20, and worsening in 1/20
Miele et al,[44] 2009	DR, R, C 8 wk	VSL3 (weight-based dosing) n = 19	Placebo n = 10	Corticosteroids, immunsuppresants, mesalamine	Remission achieved in 92% of probiotic-treated patients
Huynh et al,[43] 2009	O	VSL3 (weight-based dosing) n = 18	None	Patients were failing standard ulcerative colitis induction therapy	Remission achieved in 56% of probiotic treated-patients
Sood et al,[38] 2009	DB, R, C 12 wk	VSL3 (3.6 × 10⁹ CFU) n = 77	Placebo n = 70	Oral mesalamine and immunosuppressants	43% Achieved remission in probiotic group ($P<.001$)
Tursi et al,[39] 2010	DB, R, C 8 wk	VSL3 (3.6 × 10⁹ CFU) n = 71	Placebo n = 73	5-ASA or immunosuppressants	Remission achieved in 48% for the probiotic group
Ishikawa et al,[48] 2011	R, C 1 y	B breve strain Yakult (3 × 10⁹ CFU) and galacto-oligosaccharide (5.5 g) n = 21	Placebo n = 20	Salazosulfapyridine, mesalamine, steroids	Endoscopic score was significantly reduced in probiotic group compared with baseline ($P<.05$)
Ulcerative colitis: maintenance of remission					
Kruis et al,[49] 1997	DB, DD, R 3 mo	E coli Nissle 1917 (CFU >10¹⁰) n = 50	Mesalazine (1.6 g) n = 53	None	NSD for relapse rates, CAI scores, global assessment

Study	Design	Probiotic	Comparator	Additional therapy	Outcome
Rembacken et al,[42] 1999	DB, R, C 1 y	E coli Nissle 1917 (CFU > 10^10) n = 39	Mesalamine (1.6 g) n = 44	Prednisolone (tapered to nil over 4 mo)	NSD
Venturi et al,[85] 1999	O 1 y	VSL3 (1 × 10^12 CFU) n = 20	None	None	75% Maintained clinical and endoscopic remission
Ishikawa et al,[51] 2003	R, C 1 y	BFM n = 11	Placebo n = 10	Salazosulfapyridine, mesalazine, and steroids	Reduced exacerbation of symptoms ($P<.01$)
Cui et al,[86] 2004	DB, C 8 mo	BIFICO (1.26 g) (1 × 10^7 CFU) n = 15	Placebo n = 15	Sulphasalazine and glucocorticoids	$P<.01$ Where 93% of placebo relapsed vs 20% of active treatment group
Kruis et al,[50] 2004	DB, R, C 1 y	E coli Nissle 1917 (2.5–25 × 10^9 CFU) n = 162	Mesalamine (1.6 g) n = 165	None	As effective as mesalamine at maintaining remission (SE, $P = .003$)
Zocco et al,[53] 2006	O 1 y	L rhamnosus GG (1.8 × 10^10 CFU) n = 65	Mesalazine (2.4 g) n = 60 Mesalazine and LGG n = 62	None	NSD in relapse rates at 12 months; but probiotic more effective than mesalazine for prolonging duration of remission ($P<.05$)
Wildt et al,[54] 2011	DB, R, C 1 y	L acidophilus La-5 and B animalis and Lactis BB n = 20	Placebo n = 12	None	Insignificant number of patients achieved remission ($P = .37$)

Abbreviations: B infantis, B infantis 356,2; BFM, commercial product containing Yakult live strains of B breve, B bifidum, and L acidophilus YIT 0168; BIFICO, commercial probiotic capsule containing E terococci, Bifidobacteria, and Lactobacilli triple therapy; C, controlled; CAI, clinical activity index; DB, double blind; L acidophilus, L casei, L delbrueckii subsp bulgaricus, L plantarum, and Streptococcus salivarius subsp thermophilus; NSD, no significant difference; O, open label; R, randomized; SE, significant equivalence; VSL3, commercial mixture containing B longum, B infantis, and B breve.

[5-ASA], 6-mercaptopurine, azathioprine, and antidiarrheal agents) for 6 weeks, evaluating for the presence of probiotic bacteria in tissue samples, as well as UCDAI as an intent-to-treat analysis. This analysis demonstrated that remission was achieved in 53% (n = 18) of patients; response in 24% (n = 8) of patients; no response in 9% (n = 3) of patients; worsening in 9% (n = 3) of patients; and 5% (n = 2) did not have final sigmodmioscopic assessment. This yielded a combined induction of remission/response rate of 77%. Some components of the VSL3 bacteria were identified in 3 patients in remission. No adverse events were identified.

A Japanese study[41] investigated BIO-THREE probiotics (each tablet containing 2 mg of *Streptococcus faecalis*, 10 mg *Clostridium butyricum*, and 10 mg *Bacillus mesentericus*) in an open-label study of 23 patients with mild to moderate distal ulcerative colitis, which was refractory to medical therapy (oral mesalamine, sulfasalazine, 6-mercaptopurine, and mesalamine enema). For 4 weeks, 9 tablets were administered daily. The UCDAI scores were evaluated and fecal microflora were identified by terminal restriction fragment length polymorphism analysis. Remission was observed in 45% (9/20) of patients; response (decrease in UCDAI ≥ 3 but final score ≥ 3) in 10% (2/20); no response in 40% (8/20); and worsening in 5% (1/20). There was an overall increase in fecal bifidobacteria counts.

An early single-center, randomized, double-dummy study investigated induction of remission in 116 patients with ulcerative colitis randomized to either standard mesalazine therapy or *E coli* Nissle 1917. After a run-in course of tapering prednisolone for moderate to severe disease as well as oral gentamicin for existing microbial floral suppression, no significant differences in induction rates at 4 months were identified (75% and 68% in each group, respectively).[42] Nevertheless, this study was not powered for equivalence.

The use of probiotics in pediatric populations has demonstrated similar encouraging results. For example, an open-label trial using VSL3 twice daily in 18 eligible pediatric patients (ages 3–17) for 8 weeks was completed. Patients were evaluated by the simple clinical colitis activity index and the Mayo ulcerative colitis endoscopic score as well as various serologic and histologic profiling, completed at weeks 0 and 8. This trial demonstrated induction of remission in 56% of subjects (n = 10), response in 6% (n = 1), and no change or worse in 39% of subjects (n = 7).[43] Five patients withdrew due to lack of response to therapy.

Likewise, in a small Italian pediatric trial using VSL3,[44] 29 patients (mean age 9.8 years, range 1.7–16.1 years) with newly diagnosed ulcerative colitis, were randomized to receive VSL3 (weight-based dose, range 450–1800 billion bacteria/d) or placebo. Concomitant steroid induction treatment, consisting of oral methylprednisolone (1 mg/kg/d, maximum 40 mg/d) and oral mesalamine maintenance treatment (50 mg/kg/d), was permitted. The Lichtiger colitis activity index as well as a physician's global assessment measured disease activity. Follow-up occurred at 0, 6, and 12 months as well as whenever relapse occurred. Remission was achieved in 13 patients (92.8%) in the VSL3 group whereas 4 patients (36.4%) treated with placebo and IBD therapy had successful induction of remission (P<.001).

A Cochrane review was recently performed to delineate the role of probiotics in the induction of remission in ulcerative colitis.[45] The objectives of this review were to analyze and compare the efficacy of probiotics versus placebo or standard medical treatment (eg, corticosteroids, sulfasalazine, or 5-ASA agents) for the induction of remission in active ulcerative colitis. In addition, secondary outcome evaluation included (1) proportion of patients achieving disease improvement, (2) steroid withdrawal, (3) biochemical markers of inflammation, (4) histology scores, (5) progression to surgery, (6) clinical scores, (7) symptomatic severity (stool frequency orabdominal pain), (8) quality-of-life scores, (9) time to remission/improvement, and (10) withdrawal due to adverse events. From a total of 119 references reviewed, 4 randomized controlled trials met the inclusion criteria whereas 2 were excluded. A formal meta-analysis was not performed due to heterogeneity in probiotic types, methodology, and outcomes. The results of this review showed that none of the studies included demonstrated any meaningful differences in remission induction rates in probiotic-treated cohorts compared with placebo or other comparator groups. The investigators concluded, "Conventional therapy combined with a probiotic does not improve overall remission rates in patients with mild to moderate ulcerative colitis." With respect to safety concerns, however, one of the studies included showed that there was no statistically significant difference in the incidence of adverse events, between a group treated with probiotics and the placebo group (relative risk [RR] 0.75; 95% CI, 0.3–1.88).

In keeping with the Cochrane review, a meta-analysis performed by Sang and colleagues[46] selected 13 randomized control trials that studied the efficacy of probiotics in the induction and maintenance of remission in ulcerative colitis. Seven of the trials examined induction of remission rates in 219 patients who received probiotics as an auxiliary therapy compared with 180 patients treated with placebo or standard therapy. Again, there was no statistically significant difference in the overall induction of remission rates between the 2 groups, although the investigators concluded that the results were subject to heterogeneous bias. Furthermore, heterogeneity was also identified in a subgroup analysis with respect to probiotic type and disease severity (mild, middle, or active disease) and for treatment of less than 12 months in duration.

Optimizing the effects of probiotic organisms, Furrie and colleagues[47] sought to evaluate the effect of the combination of probiotics and prebiotics (synbiotics) containing *Bifidobacterium longum* and Synergy 1 (6 g of prebiotic fructo-oligosaccharide/inulin mix) in a double-blind randomized controlled trial using 18 patients (N = 9, study group) with active ulcerative colitis for a period of 1 month. The patients' standard therapy at the time of entry into the study remained unchanged (steroids and/or immunosuppressants and/or 5-ASA). The results demonstrated a systemic anti-inflammatory response with a decrease in serum TNF-α ($P = .018$), interleukin 1 ($P = .023$), and mRNA levels of defensins 2 and 4. Nevertheless there were no significant differences in sigmoidoscopy or clinical disease activity indices.

Similarly, Ishikawa and colleagues[48] in a randomized controlled trial evaluated 41 patients with mild to moderate ulcerative colitis administered synbiotics. This trial used a *B breve* strain; Yakult (9×10^9 CFU/g) was administered in divided doses 3 times daily in combination with galacto-oligogosaccharide (5.5 g once daily, for 1 year) in comparison to placebo. Both groups were allowed standard medical therapy. Endoscopic evaluation of disease activity was performed at 1 year as well as evaluation of a colonic lavage solution for myeloperoxidase activity. Mean endoscopic disease activity score of patients receiving synbiotics decreased significantly ($P<.05$) relative to placebo. Furthermore, myeloperoxidase activity in the treatment group significantly decreased ($P<.05$).

In summary, the existing evidence does not support the broad use of probiotics in the induction of remission in patients with active ulcerative colitis. Not all probiotics are the same and randomized controlled trials of each individual probiotic preparation are required to determine its efficacy. Nevertheless, emerging data from 2 double-blind randomized controlled trials and 3 open-label trials with the probiotic preparation VSL3 are supportive of its efficacy in the induction of remission of ulcerative colitis. In addition, a single trial with *E coli* Nissle 1917 suggests it may be as effective as mesalamine. These trials, however, were underpowered to be statistically confirmatory.

Probiotics and ulcerative colitis: induction of remission recall points

- Currently, there are insufficient data to support the broad use of probiotics in inducing remission in patients with acute ulcerative colitis.
- Nevertheless, underpowered randomized controlled trials with the probiotic preparation VSL3 have demonstrated its efficacy over placebo in the induction of remission, and *E coli* Nissle 1917 may be as effective as mesalamine.

Maintenance of remission

Kruis and colleagues[49] first examined remission maintenance in ulcerative colitis in 120 patients who previously achieved a mesalamine-induced remission. These patients were subsequently randomized to 1600 mg of mesalamine or *E coli* Nissle 1917. Similar efficacy was identified in both groups at 3 months, with 89% and 84% of the respective groups in remission. Subsequently, the same investigators completed a multicenter, randomized noninferiority trial comparing mesalamine (1600 mg daily) versus *E coli* Nissle 1917 in 327 patients over a 12-month period.[50] *E coli* Nissle was found statistically noninferior ($P = .013$), with relapse rates of 34% in the mesalamine group and 36% in the *E coli* Nissle 1917 group.

A prospective, noninferiority trial by Rembacken found similar results in a study comparing oral mesalamine (1600 mg daily) to *E coli* Nissle 1917 in 116 patients.[42] After 12 months, 25% and 26% of the respective groups were found in remission. Furthermore, the rates of remission were found similar to known rates of remission achieved with placebo.

In a randomized, placebo-controlled trial in 21 patients, Ishikawa and colleagues[51] examined the effect of fermented milk, which contained live *Bifidobacteria* and *L acidophilus* in patients with quiescent ulcerative colitis. Clinical remission was sustained over 1 year in 73% of patients taking the probiotic versus 10% in the placebo arm ($P = .0184$). No endoscopic differences, however, were noted.

Shanahan and von Wright[52] compared *L salivarius* subsp *salivarius* UCC118, *B infatis* 35,624 (1×10^9 CFU/d) or placebo for 1 year in patients with ulcerative colitis in clinical remission (n = 157 patients). There was no significant difference in time to relapse when placebo was compared with either treatment arm. Nevertheless, the probiotics demonstrated an anti-inflammatory effect.

Another prospective randomized trial by Zocco and colleagues[53] compared *Lactobacillus* GG (1.8×10^9 viable bacteria/d) to delayed-released mesalamine (2400 mg daily) or both in 187 patients with ulcerative colitis. Based on UCDAI scores, relapse rates were similar at 6 months ($P = .44$) and at 12 months ($P = .77$) in all 3 groups, *Lactobacillus* GG did prolong relapse-free time more effectively than mesalamine ($P < .05$).

A recent trial out of Denmark sought to investigate the clinical effects of a combination of *L acidophilus* La-5 and *B animalis* subsp *lactis* BB (Probio-Tec AB-25) in maintenance of remission in a randomized double-blind placebo-controlled trial in 32 patients with ulcerative colitis.[54] These patients included those with left-sided ulcerative colitis in remission, including proctitis. All patients had at least one relapse within the year preceding the trial. Twenty patients received Probio-Tec AB-25 whereas 12 received placebo. After 1 year of treatment, 5 patients (25%) in the Priobio-Tec AB-25 group and 1 patient (8%) in the placebo group were in remission ($P = .37$). The median times to relapse were 125.5 days (11–391 days) and 104 days (28–369 days), respectively ($P = .683$). Although encouraging, the study was of small size and did not reach statistical significance.

A Cochrane database review in 2011 was performed by Naidoo and colleagues[55] to evaluate the role of probiotics in the maintenance of remission in patients with ulcerative colitis. Four studies (n = 587) with study duration from 3 to 12 months were included. There were no statistically significant differences between the probiotic-treated and mesalamine-treated patients (40.1% vs 34.1%, respectively; 3 studies; 555 patients; odds ratio [OR] 1.33; 95% CI, 0.94–1.90) and in adverse events (26% vs 24%, respectively; 2 studies; 430 patients; OR 1.21; 95% CI, 0.80–1.84). The investigators identified risk of bias due to lack of blinding and incomplete outcome data (2 studies), and unclear methods of allocation in all 4 studies.

In summary, there is adequately powered randomized controlled trial evidence to support that *E coli* Nissle 1917 is as effective as mesalamine in maintaining remission in patients with mild to moderate ulcerative colitis. Not all probiotics are the same and randomized controlled trials of each individual probiotic preparation are required to determine their efficacy.

Probiotics and ulcerative colitis: maintenance of remission recall point
- *E coli* Nissle 1917 is as effective as mesalamine in maintaining remission in patients with mild to moderate ulcerative colitis.

Pouchitis

In patients with ulcerative colitis in whom medical management fails, total colectomy and construction of an ileal pouch–anal anastomosis (IPAA) is the surgical approach of choice (**Table 2**). More than half of these patients develop inflammation of the pouch, leading to pouchitis, with symptoms of pain, diarrhea, and often fecal incontinence. A summary of the clinical trials that examined probiotics in the induction and maintenance of remission in pouchitis is in **Table 2**.

Induction and maintenance of remission

An early, randomized, double-blind, placebo-controlled trial by Gionchetti and colleagues[56] demonstrated successful maintenance of remission with probiotics in 40 patients. These patients first underwent a successful induction of remission of their pouchitis with antibiotics and then were randomized to VSL3 or placebo. After 9 months, 85% of the VSL3-treated patients versus 0% of those on placebo were in remission. Relapse of pouchitis occurred within 3 months in those patients who had their VSL3 discontinued.

In a follow-up, double-blind, placebo-controlled trial Gionchetti sought to examine primary prevention of pouchitis in patients who had recently undergone an IPAA operation.[57] In 40 consecutive patients, immediately after IPAA construction, 20 were randomized to VSL3 (9 × 10^9 CFU/d whereas 20 received placebo for 12 months. Every 3 months, clinical, endoscopic, and histologic evaluations were performed. At 12 months, 90% of VSL3-treated patients and 60% of placebo-treated patients were in remission (log-rank test, z = 2.273; $P<.05$).

Similar to the early trial by Gionchetti, Mimura and colleagues[58] also examined the maintenance of remission after inducing pouchitis into remission with antibiotics. The trial compared VSL3 to placebo in a double-blind randomized controlled study. Remission rates after 12 months were 85% in the VSL3-treated group versus 6% in the placebo-treated arm, supporting the previous findings by Gionchetti.

In an open-label trial, using *Lactobacillus* GG, Gosselink and colleagues[59] also demonstrated the ability of another probiotic to maintain remission after induction of pouchitis remission with antibiotics. In this study, 93% of patients treated with *Lactobacillus* GG were in remission at 12 months. Divergent from this maintenance of remission data with *Lactobacillus* GG, Kuisma and colleagues[60] did not find *Lactobacillus* GG able to induce remission in patients with acute pouchitis. Over a 3-month period,

Table 2
Evidence for the effect of probiotic treatments in pouchitis

First Author, Year	Design Duration	Group (dose/d) Probiotic	Comparator	Concomitant Therapy	Results
Pouchitis: induction of remission					
Kuisma et al,[60] 2003	DB, R, C 3 mo	Lactobacillus GG (1 × 10^10 CFU) n = 10	Placebo n = 10	Not indicated	No difference in pouch disease activity index
Laake et al,[87] 2004	O 4 wk	L acidophilus and B lactis– fermented milk (500 mL) n = 51	None	Loperamide	Improved pouch disease activity index; no difference in histology
Pronio et al,[36] 2008	O 1 y	VSL3 n = 31	None	None	Reduction in pouch disease activity index
Pouchitis: maintenance of remission					
Gionchetti et al,[88] 2000	DB, R, C 9 mo	VSL3 (6 g) n = 20	Placebo n = 20	None	Increased duration of remission (P<.001)
Gionchetti et al,[57] 2003	DB, R, C 1 y	VSL3 (1 × 10^11 CFU) n = 20	Placebo n = 20	None	Increased duration of remission (P<.05)
Gosselink et al,[59] 2004	R, C 3 y	L rhamnosus GG (CFU > 10^10) n = 78	Placebo n = 39	Not indicated	Increased duration of remission (P = .011)
Mimura et al,[58] 2004	DB, R, C 1 y	VSL3 (6 g) n = 20	Placebo n = 16	Not indicated	Increased duration of remission (P<.0001)

Abbreviations: C, controlled; DB, double blind; L acidophilus, L casei, L delbrueckii subsp bulgaricus, L plantarum, and Streptococcus salivarius subsp thermophilus; O, open label; R, randomized; VSL3, commercial mixture containing B longum, B infantis, and B breve.

only 40% of patients with acute pouchitis treated with *Lactobacillus* GG were colonized with the *Lactobacillus* GG and no clinical benefit was realized in the treatment group compared with the placebo group.

Given the efficacy of VSL3 in maintenance of remission of pouchitis, studies have been performed to document changes in mucosal inflammation and characterize the associated changes in the mucosal and systemic immune systems and luminal microbial profiles. An Italian study by Pronio and colleagues[36] examined the effects of VSL3 in 31 IPAA patients in an open-label trial lasting 1 year. This demonstrated an expansion in CD4+ T lymphocytes expressing CD25 (CD4+ CD25 high), CD4+ latency-associated peptide (CD4+ LAP), interleukin-1β in peripheral blood mononuclear cells, and mucosal biopsies, all indices demonstrating enhanced anti-inflammatory effects. Accordingly, patients experienced a reduction in their pouch activity index. Studies of pouch biodiversity have shown reduction in both species type and absolute colony count in those patients who have undergone IPAA for ulcerative colitis when compared with those who have undergone IPAA for familial adenomatous polyposis.[61] In addition, in a murine model of colitis induced by 2,4,6-trinitrobenzenesulfonic acid, VSL3 reduced mucosal inflammation in association with a reduction in biodiversity.[62]

In summary, there are randomized controlled studies supporting VSL3 and *Lactobacillus* GG in the maintenance of remission of pouchits after IPAA or antibiotic-induced remission, respectively. Not all probiotics are the same and randomized controlled trials of each individual probiotic preparation are required to determine its efficacy.

Probiotics and pouchitis: recall points
- Probiotics have been shown effective in maintenance of remission of patients with pouchitis.

Crohn Disease

Induction of remission
Table 3 summarizes the clinical trials that examined probiotics in the induction and maintenance of remission in Crohn disease.

A recent clinical trial by Steed and colleagues[63] evaluated mucosal TNF-α levels and remission rates in 35 patients with Crohn disease, who were randomized to either placebo or a synbiotic comprising *B longum* and Synergy 1 while on concurrent immunomodulation or immunosuppression. There were significant improvements in mean CDAI scores in the synbiotic group (start 219 ± 74.6, finish 147 ± 74; $P = .020$) but not in the placebo group (start 249 ± 79.4, finish 233 ± 155; $P = .810$) after 6 months. Similar improvements in mean histologic scores in the synbiotic group ($P = .018$) were also seen over the same time. A significant initial reduction in mucosal TNF-α levels ($P = .041$) at 3 months was not maintained at 6 months.

These encouraging data, however, have not been the rule. In 2008, Butterworth and colleagues[64] completed a Cochrane review of the role of probiotics in the induction of remission of active Crohn disease and confirmed that a favorable therapeutic response in these patients remains to be seen. Included in this analysis were small open-label trials because no randomized placebo-controlled trials existed. In 2004, Schultz and colleagues[65] used *Lactobacillus* GG in patients with active Crohn disease who were initially treated with concurrent steroids and antibiotics for 1 week and then randomized to receive either *Lactobacillus* GG or placebo. Of the 5 of 11 patients who completed the trial, the time to relapse was similar between treatment and the placebo groups (12 wk vs 16 wk, $P = .5$). Another open-label trial by Fujimori and colleagues[66] in 2007 showed improvement in CDAI scores in 7 of 10 patients treated with

Table 3
Induction and maintenance of remission in Crohn disease: a summary of evidence investigating the effect of probiotic treatments

First Author, Date	Design Duration	Group (dose/d)		Concomitant Therapy	Results
		Probiotic	Comparator		
Crohn disease: induction of remission					
Gupta et al,[68] 2000	O, 6 mo	LGG (2 × 10^{10} CFU) n = 4	None	Prednisone, immunomodulatory agents, metronidazole	Improved CDAI scores compared with baseline (P<.05)
McCarthy et al,[67] 2001	O, N/A	L salivarius UCC118	None	N/A	Improved CDAI scores
Schultz et al,[65] 2004	DB, R, C, 6 mo	LGG (2 × 10^9 CFU) n = 5	Placebo n = 6	Ciprofloxacin, metronidazole, corticosteroids	NSD
Fujimori et al,[66] 2007	O, 13 ± 4.5 mo	B breve (3 × 10^{10} CFU), L casei (3 × 10^{10} CFU), B longum (1.5 × 10^{10} CFU), Psyllium (9.9 g) n = 10	None	Aminosalicylate, prednisolone, home enteral nutrition	Improved CDAI and IOIBD scores compared with baseline (255–136, P = .009, and 3.5–2.1, P = .03, respectively). 60% (6/10) achieved remission
Steed et al,[63] 2010	DB, R, C, 6 mo	B longum (4 × 10^{11} CFU) and Synergy 1 (12 g) n = 13	Placebo n = 11	Steroids and/or immunomodulators	Reductions in TNF-α expression and CDAI at 3 months (P = .041)
Crohn disease: maintenance of remission					
Malchow et al,[89] 1997	DB, R, C, 1 y	E coli Nissle 1917 (5 × 10^{10} CFU) n = 16	Placebo n = 12	Prednisolone	NSD
Guslandi et al,[69] 2000	R, C, 6 mo	S boulardii (1 g) and mesalamine (2 g) n = 16	Mesalamine (3 g) n = 16	Not indicated	Increased duration of remission (P<.05)

Study	Design	Treatment	Placebo	Concomitant medication	Outcome
Prantera et al,[72] 2002	DB, R, C 1 y	LGG (1.2 × 10^10 CFU) n = 23	Placebo n = 22	Loperamide, cholestyramine	NSD
Bousvaros et al,[71] 2005	DB, R, C 2 y	LGG (4 × 10^10 CFU) n = 39	Placebo n = 36	Aminosalicylates, 6-mercaptopurine, azathioprine, corticosteroids	NSD
Marteau et al,[73] 2006	DB, R, C 6 mo	L johnsonii LA1, Nestle (2 × 10^9 CFU) n = 43	Placebo n = 47	Loperamide, cholestyramine, corticosteroids tapered to nil by wk 3	NSD for endoscopic scores *Dropout rate (n = 8)
Chermesh et al,[77] 2007	DB, R, C 2 y	Synbiotic 2000 n = 7	Placebo n = 2	Not indicated	NSD regarding postoperative recurrence of symptoms *High dropout rate (n = 21)
Vilela et al,[70] 2008	R, C 3 mo	S boulardii (1.2 × 10^9 CFU) n = 14	Placebo n = 17	Mesalamine, immunosuppressants, thalidomide	Improved intestinal permeability vs placebo (P = .0005)

Abbreviations: C, controlled; DB, double blind; LGG, L rhamnosus GG; N/A, not available; NSD, no significant difference; O, open label; R, randomized; *, special note.

a combination of *Lactobacillus* and *Bifidobacterium* species. Another uncontrolled open-label trial in 2001 also showed an improvement in CDAI scores in patients with Crohn disease treated with *L salivarius* UCC118.[67] In 2000, Gupta and colleagues[68] evaluated the possible benefits of twice-daily dosing of *Lactobacillus* GG in a 6-month open-label trial in 4 pediatric patients with Crohn disease taking concomitant glucocorticoid and/or immunomodulator therapy.[68] By the end of the first week, the Pediatric Crohn Disease Activity Index (PCDAI) score had improved and this effect was maintained throughout the study period. At 4 weeks, 3 patients had a PCDAI score of less than 10 (median PCDAI score = 5, range 0–12.5), 73% lower than base-line. Glucocorticoid tapering was achieved in 3 patients, whereas 3 patients experienced clinical relapses, 4 to 12 weeks after discontinuing the probiotic.

In summary, there is no evidence for the use of probiotics in induction of remission in Crohn disease. The existing clinical trials are small and open label. Not all probiotics are the same and randomized controlled trials of each individual probiotic preparation are required to determine its efficacy.

Probiotics and Crohn disease: induction of remission recall points
- There is insufficient evidence to support probiotic use in inducing remission in patients with Crohn disease.

Maintenance of medically induced remission

In an early small trial[69] using *Saccharomyces boulardii*, 32 patients with Crohn disease were randomized to either mesalamine (1 g 3 times a day) or mesalamine (1 g 2 times a day) in addition to a preparation of *S boulardii* (1 g daily). Clinical remission was observed in 94% and 62% of patients, respectively ($P = .04$).

Given that mucosal permeability is increased in Crohn disease, Vilela and colleagues[70] examined the effects of *S boulardii* or placebo in 34 patients with Crohn disease in remission, measuring intestinal permeability with lactulose/mannitol ratios. Again, current therapeutic regimen remained unaltered. In the placebo group, there was worsening of the intestinal permeability with an increase in the lactulose/mannitol ratio by 0.004 ± 0.010 ($P = .12$) at the end of the third month. In contrast, in the *S boulardii*–treated group, there was an improvement in intestinal permeability, with a decrease in the lactulose/mannitol ratio by 0.008 ± 0.006 ($P = .0005$). Complete normalization of intestinal permeability, however, was not achieved.

Most studies in Crohn disease, however, are not supportive of a probiotic effect. Bousvaros and colleagues[71] found no difference in relapse rates in 75 pediatric Crohn disease patients receiving either 2×10^{10} CFU of *L rhamnosus* GG or placebo over a period of 24 months (71% vs 83%, respectively). Similarly, other studies have demonstrated results for *Lactobacillus* that are in keeping with this.[72,73]

A Cochrane review in 2006[74] failed to demonstrate any benefit for probiotics as maintenance therapy in patients with Crohn disease; however, the investigators observed that due to low patient enrollment, statistical power may have been affected. In 2008, Rahimi and colleagues[75] conducted a meta-analysis, which included 8 randomized controlled trials evaluating the role of probiotics in the maintenance of remission and in Crohn disease. No significant differences were noted for either clinical relapse (OR = 0.92 [0.52–1.62]) or endoscopic relapse (OR = 0.97 [0.54–1.78]).

In 2009, Shen and colleagues,[76] in a meta-analysis, evaluated *Lactobacillus* species with respect to efficacy and adverse events as maintenance therapy in patients with Crohn disease. They included 6 trials (359 patients) comparing *Lactobacilli* with placebo; the RR of clinical relapse rate was 1.15 (95% CI, 0.90–1.48) and the RR of endoscopic relapse rate was 1.31 (95% CI, 0.57–3.00), whereas the pooled RR of adverse events was 0.83 (95% CI, 0.61–1.12). They suggested that *L rhamnosus* GG might actually increase the relapse rate in patients with Crohn disease.

In summary, there is no evidence for the use of probiotics in maintenance of medically induced remission in Crohn disease. The existing clinical trials are small and open label. Not all probiotics are the same and randomized controlled trials of each individual probiotic preparation are required to determine its efficacy.

Probiotics and Crohn disease: maintenance of medically induced remission recall points

- There is insufficient evidence to support probiotic use in maintenance of medically induced remission in patients with Crohn disease.

Maintenance of surgically induced remission

There remains to be definitive evidence to support the use of probiotic organisms as maintenance therapy in patients with Crohn disease who have had remission induced via surgical means. Prantera and colleagues[72] used *Lactobacillus* GG in 45 patients versus placebo, administered within 10 days postoperatively to patients undergoing intestinal resection for their Crohn disease. At 12 months, no significant endoscopic or clinical differences were realized between the 2 groups. Furthermore, Marteau and colleagues[73] performed a randomized, placebo-controlled trial comparing *Lactobacillus johnsonii* LA1 (2×10^9 CFU/d) to placebo and found no clinical or endoscopic differences (98 patients) at 6 months.

A meta-analysis in 2009 by Doherty[78] confirmed the ineffectiveness of probiotics versus placebo in the control of surgically induced remission in patients with Crohn disease: RR of clinical recurrence with any probiotic = 1.41 (95% CI, 0.59–3.36) and RR of endoscopic recurrence = 0.98 (95% CI, 0.74–1.29).

In hopes of improving the efficacy of probiotics, Chermesh and colleagues[77] sought to evaluate a mixture of 4 prebiotics (nondigestible foodstuffs used to stimulate the activity of bacteria within the gastrointestinal tract) and 4 probiotics (Synbiotic 2000) to placebo in postoperative patients with Crohn disease. Again, no discernible endoscopic or clinical differences were noted.

In summary, there is little evidence to support the use of probiotics in the setting of postoperative patient with Crohn disease in hopes of preventing clinical or endoscopic relapse.

Probiotics and surgical patients with Crohn disease: maintenance of surgically induced remission recall points

- There are insufficient data to support probiotic use in maintaining surgically induced remission in patients with Crohn disease in the postoperative state

SUMMARY

The presence of a diverse microbial population within the gastrointestinal tract and the changes that occur during IBD provide reasonable support for the use of probiotic organisms in the treatment of ulcerative colitis, pouchitis, and Crohn disease.[79] Double-blind, randomized controlled studies support the therapeutic role of some, but not all, probiotics in the treatment of ulcerative colitis and pouchitis but not yet Crohn disease. Nonetheless, challenges remain. Not all probiotics are the same and thus properly powered and controlled clinical trials are needed for each probiotic preparation before it can be accepted as a therapeutic modality. There does not seem to be a "class" effect for probiotics. Despite this, the human gastrointestinal tract represents a dynamic environment for the microbe, with changes in host anatomy, physiology, and disease states affecting microbe diversity and, in turn, microbe diversity affecting the host and disease states.[80] There is much to be done in the field of probiotic research, both at the microbial and mechanism of action levels and also within the clinical trial realm. Specifically, future large scale prospective trials are required to move beyond the prevalence of current small uncontrolled trials with probiotics. For probiotic treatment to advance and become mainstream, they need to be seen and treated as clinically significant pharmacotherapeutic agents, with appropriate consideration given to their efficacy and safety profiles.

REFERENCES

1. Rawsthorne P, Clara I, Graff LA, et al. The manitoba inflammatory bowel disease cohort study: a prospective longitudinal evaluation of the use of complementary and alternative medicine services and products. Gut 2012;61(4):521–7.
2. Abraham C, Medzhitov R. Interactions between the host innate immune system and microbes in inflammatory bowel disease. Gastroenterology 2011;140(6):1729–37.
3. Chassaing B, Darfeuille-Michaud A. The commensal microbiota and enteropath-ogens in the pathogenesis of inflammatory bowel diseases. Gastroenterology 2011;140(6):1720–8.
4. Mercenier A, Pavan S, Pot B. Probiotics as biotherapeutic agents: present knowl-edge and future prospects. Curr Pharm Des 2003;9(2):175–91.
5. Sazawal S, Hiremath G, Dhingra U, et al. Efficacy of probiotics in prevention of acute diarrhoea: a meta-analysis of masked, randomised, placebo-controlled trials. Lancet Infect Dis 2006;6(6):374–82.
6. Allen SJ, Martinez EG, Gregorio GV, et al. Probiotics for treating acute infectious diarrhoea. Cochrane Database Syst Rev 2010;(11):CD003048.
7. Brenner DM, Moeller MJ, Chey WD, et al. The utility of probiotics in the treatment of irritable bowel syndrome: a systematic review. Am J Gastroenterol 2009; 104(4):1033–49 [Quiz: 1050].
8. Deshpande G, Rao S, Patole S, et al. Updated meta-analysis of probiotics for pre-venting necrotizing enterocolitis in preterm neonates. Pediatrics 2010;125(5): 921–30.
9. Bajaj JS, Saeian K, Christensen KM, et al. Probiotic yogurt for the treatment of minimal hepatic encephalopathy. Am J Gastroenterol 2008;103(7):1707–15.
10. Eckburg PB, Bik EM, Bernstein CN, et al. Diversity of the human intestinal micro-bial flora. Science 2005;308(5728):1635–8.
11. Dominguez-Bello MG, Costello EK, Contreras M, et al. Delivery mode shapes the acquisition and structure of the initial microbiota across multiple body habitats in newborns. Proc Natl Acad Sci U S A 2010;107(26):11971–5.
12. Palmer C, Bik EM, DiGiulio DB, et al. Development of the human infant intestinal microbiota. PLoS Biol 2007;5(7):e177.
13. Penders J, Thijs C, Vink C, et al. Factors influencing the composition of the intes-tinal microbiota in early infancy. Pediatrics 2006;118(2):511–21.
14. Claesson MJ, Cusack S, O'Sullivan O, et al. Composition, variability, and temporal stability of the intestinal microbiota of the elderly. Proc Natl Acad Sci U S A 2011;108(Suppl 1):4586–91.
15. D'Haens GR, Geboes K, Peeters M, et al. Early lesions of recurrent Crohn's disease caused by infusion of intestinal contents in excluded ileum. Gastroenter-ology 1998;114(2):262–7.
16. Nishikawa J, Kudo T, Sakata S, et al. Diversity of mucosa-associated microbiota in active and inactive ulcerative colitis. Scand J Gastroenterol 2009;44(2):180–6.

17. Willing BP, Dicksved J, Halfvarson J, et al. A pyrosequencing study in twins shows that gastrointestinal microbial profiles vary with inflammatory bowel disease phenotypes. Gastroenterology 2010;139(6):1844–1854.e1.

18. Sokol H, Pigneur B, Watterlot L, et al. Faecalibacterium prausnitzii is an anti-inflammatory commensal bacterium identified by gut microbiota analysis of Crohn disease patients. Proc Natl Acad Sci U S A 2008;105(43):16731–6.

19. Swidsinski A, Ladhoff A, Pernthaler A, et al. Mucosal flora in inflammatory bowel disease. Gastroenterology 2002;122(1):44–54.

20. Manichanh C, Rigottier-Gois L, Bonnaud E, et al. Reduced diversity of faecal microbiota in Crohn's disease revealed by a metagenomic approach. Gut 2006; 55(2):205–11.

21. Neut C, Bulois P, Desreumaux P, et al. Changes in the bacterial flora of the neo-terminal ileum after ileocolonic resection for Crohn's disease. Am J Gastroenterol 2002;97(4):939–46.

22. Swidsinski A, Loening-Baucke V, Theissig F, et al. Comparative study of the intestinal mucus barrier in normal and inflamed colon. Gut 2007;56(3):343–50.

23. Martin HM, Campbell BJ, Hart CA, et al. Enhanced Escherichia coli adherence and invasion in Crohn's disease and colon cancer. Gastroenterology 2004; 127(1):80–93.

24. Mondot S, Kang S, Furet JP, et al. Highlighting new phylogenetic specificities of Crohn's disease microbiota. Inflamm Bowel Dis 2011;17(1):185–92.

25. Seksik P, Rigottier-Gois L, Gramet G, et al. Alterations of the dominant faecal bacterial groups in patients with Crohn's disease of the colon. Gut 2003;52(2):237–42.

26. Sartor RB. Does Mycobacterium avium subspecies paratuberculosis cause Crohn's disease? Gut 2005;54(7):896–8.

27. Bentley RW, Keenan JI, Gearry RB, et al. Incidence of Mycobacterium avium subspecies paratuberculosis in a population-based cohort of patients with Crohn's disease and control subjects. Am J Gastroenterol 2008;103(5):1168–72.

28. Saebo A, Vik E, Lange OJ, et al. Inflammatory bowel disease associated with Yersinia enterocolitica O:3 infection. Eur J Intern Med 2005;16(3):176–82.

29. Man SM, Zhang L, Day AS, et al. Campylobacter concisus and other Campylobacter species in children with newly diagnosed Crohn's disease. Inflamm Bowel Dis 2010;16(6):1008–16.

30. Darfeuille-Michaud A, Boudeau J, Bulois P, et al. High prevalence of adherent-invasive Escherichia coli associated with ileal mucosa in Crohn's disease. Gastroenterology 2004;127(2):412–21.

31. Hotte NS, Salim SY, Tso RH, et al. Patients with inflammatory bowel disease exhibit dysregulated responses to microbial DNA. PLoS One 2012;7(5):e37932.

32. Guillemard E, Tondu F, Lacoin F, et al. Consumption of a fermented dairy product containing the probiotic Lactobacillus casei DN-114001 reduces the duration of respiratory infections in the elderly in a randomised controlled trial. Br J Nutr 2010;103(1):58–68.

33. Boge T, Remigy M, Vaudaine S, et al. A probiotic fermented dairy drink improves antibody response to influenza vaccination in the elderly in two randomised controlled trials. Vaccine 2009;27(41):5677–84.

34. Demeria DM. Interactions of Lactobacillus with the immune system. In: Ljungh AW, editor. Lactobacillus molecular biology: from genomics to probiotics. 1st edition. Sweden: Caister Academic Press; 2009. p. 206.

35. Mikelsaar M, Stsepetova J, Hutt P, et al. Intestinal Lactobacillus sp. is associated with some cellular and metabolic characteristics of blood in elderly people. Anaerobe 2010;16(3):240–6.

36. Pronio A, Montesani C, Butteroni C, et al. Probiotic administration in patients with ileal pouch-anal anastomosis for ulcerative colitis is associated with expansion of mucosal regulatory cells. Inflamm Bowel Dis 2008;14(5):662–8.

37. Lammers KM, Vergopoulos A, Babel N, et al. Probiotic therapy in the prevention of pouchitis onset: decreased interleukin-1beta, interleukin-8, and interferon-gamma gene expression. Inflamm Bowel Dis 2005;11(5):447–54.

38. Sood A, Midha V, Makharia GK, et al. The probiotic preparation, VSL#3 induces remission in patients with mild-to-moderately active ulcerative colitis. Clin Gastroenterol Hepatol 2009;7(11):1202–9, 1209.e1201.

39. Tursi A, Brandimarte G, Papa A, et al. Treatment of relapsing mild-to-moderate ulcerative colitis with the probiotic VSL#3 as adjunctive to a standard pharmaceutical treatment: a double-blind, randomized, placebo-controlled study. Am J Gastroenterol 2010;105(10):2218–27.

40. Bibiloni R, Fedorak RN, Tannock GW, et al. VSL#3 probiotic-mixture induces remission in patients with active ulcerative colitis. Am J Gastroenterol 2005;100(7):1539–46.

41. Tsuda Y, Yoshimatsu Y, Aoki H, et al. Clinical effectiveness of probiotics therapy (BIO-THREE) in patients with ulcerative colitis refractory to conventional therapy. Scand J Gastroenterol 2007;42(11):1306–11.

42. Rembacken BJ, Snelling AM, Hawkey PM, et al. Non-pathogenic Escherichia coli versus mesalazine for the treatment of ulcerative colitis: a randomised trial. Lancet 1999;354(9179):635–9.

43. Huynh HQ, deBruyn J, Guan L, et al. Probiotic preparation VSL#3 induces remission in children with mild to moderate acute ulcerative colitis: a pilot study. Inflamm Bowel Dis 2009;15(5):760–8.

44. Miele E, Pascarella F, Giannetti E, et al. Effect of a probiotic preparation (VSL#3) on induction and maintenance of remission in children with ulcerative colitis. Am J Gastroenterol 2009;104(2):437–43.

45. Mallon P, McKay D, Kirk S, et al. Probiotics for induction of remission in ulcerative colitis. Cochrane Database Syst Rev 2007;(4):CD005573.

46. Sang LX, Chang B, Zhang WL, et al. Remission induction and maintenance effect of probiotics on ulcerative colitis: a meta-analysis. World J Gastroenterol 2010;16(15):1908–15.

47. Furrie E, Macfarlane S, Kennedy A, et al. Synbiotic therapy (Bifidobacterium longum/Synergy 1) initiates resolution of inflammation in patients with active ulcerative colitis: a randomised controlled pilot trial. Gut 2005;54(2):242–9.

48. Ishikawa H, Matsumoto S, Ohashi Y, et al. Beneficial effects of probiotic bifidobacterium and galacto-oligosaccharide in patients with ulcerative colitis: a randomized controlled study. Digestion 2011;84(2):128–33.

49. Kruis W, Schutz E, Fric P, et al. Double-blind comparison of an oral Escherichia coli preparation and mesalazine in maintaining remission of ulcerative colitis. Aliment Pharmacol Ther 1997;11(5):853–8.

50. Kruis W, Fric P, Pokrotnieks J, et al. Maintaining remission of ulcerative colitis with the probiotic Escherichia coli Nissle 1917 is as effective as with standard mesalazine. Gut 2004;53(11):1617–23.

51. Ishikawa H, Akedo I, Umesaki Y, et al. Randomized controlled trial of the effect of bifidobacteria-fermented milk on ulcerative colitis. J Am Coll Nutr 2003;22(1):56–63.

52. Shanahan FG, Guaraner F, von Wright A, et al. A one year, double-blind, placebo controlled trial fo a Lactobacillus or a Bidfidobacterium probiotic for maintenance of steroid-induced remission of ulcerative colitis. Gastroenterology 2006;130(Suppl 2):A-44.

53. Zocco MA, dal Verme LZ, Cremonini F, et al. Efficacy of Lactobacillus GG in maintaining remission of ulcerative colitis. Aliment Pharmacol Ther 2006;23(11):1567–74.
54. Wildt S, Nordgaard I, Hansen U, et al. A randomised double-blind placebo-controlled trial with Lactobacillus acidophilus La-5 and Bifidobacterium animalis subsp. lactis BB-12 for maintenance of remission in ulcerative colitis. J Crohns Colitis 2011;5(2):115–21.
55. Naidoo K, Gordon M, Fagbemi AO, et al. Probiotics for maintenance of remission in ulcerative colitis. Cochrane Database Syst Rev 2011;(12):CD007443.
56. Gionchetti PA, Amadini C, Rizzello F, et al. Probiotics—role in inflammatory bowel disease. Dig Liver Dis 2002;34(Suppl 2):S58–62.
57. Gionchetti P, Rizzello F, Helwig U, et al. Prophylaxis of pouchitis onset with probiotic therapy: a double-blind, placebo-controlled trial. Gastroenterology 2003; 124(5):1202–9.
58. Mimura T, Rizzello F, Helwig U, et al. Once daily high dose probiotic therapy (VSL#3) for maintaining remission in recurrent or refractory pouchitis. Gut 2004;53(1):108–14.
59. Gosselink MP, Schouten WR, van Lieshout LM, et al. Delay of the first onset of pouchitis by oral intake of the probiotic strain Lactobacillus rhamnosus GG. Dis Colon Rectum 2004;47(6):876–84.
60. Kuisma J, Mentula S, Jarvinen H, et al. Effect of Lactobacillus rhamnosus GG on ileal pouch inflammation and microbial flora. Aliment Pharmacol Ther 2003;17(4): 509–15.
61. McLaughlin SD, Walker AW, Churcher C, et al. The bacteriology of pouchitis: a molecular phylogenetic analysis using 16S rRNA gene cloning and sequencing. Ann Surg 2010;252(1):90–8.
62. Uronis JM, Arthur JC, Keku T, et al. Gut microbial diversity is reduced by the probiotic VSL#3 and correlates with decreased TNBS-induced colitis. Inflamm Bowel Dis 2011;17(1):289–97.
63. Steed H, Macfarlane GT, Blackett KL, et al. Clinical trial: the microbiological and immunological effects of synbiotic consumption - a randomized double-blind placebo-controlled study in active Crohn's disease. Aliment Pharmacol Ther 2010;32(7):872–83.
64. Butterworth AD, Thomas AG, Akobeng AK. Probiotics for induction of remission in Crohn's disease. Cochrane Database Syst Rev 2008;(3):CD006634.
65. Schultz M, Timmer A, Herfarth HH, et al. Lactobacillus GG in inducing and maintaining remission of Crohn's disease. BMC Gastroenterol 2004;4:5.
66. Fujimori S, Tatsuguchi A, Gudis K, et al. High dose probiotic and prebiotic cotherapy for remission induction of active Crohn's disease. J Gastroenterol Hepatol 2007;22(8):1199–204.
67. McCarthy J, O'Mahony L, Dunne C. An open trial of a novel probiotic as an alternative to steroids in mild/moderately active Crohn's disease [abstract]. Gut 2001; 49(Suppl III):A2447.
68. Gupta P, Andrew H, Kirschner BS, et al. Is lactobacillus GG helpful in children with Crohn's disease? Results of a preliminary, open-label study. J Pediatr Gastroenterol Nutr 2000;31(4):453–7.
69. Guslandi M, Mezzi G, Sorghi M, et al. Saccharomyces boulardii in maintenance treatment of Crohn's disease. Dig Dis Sci 2000;45(7):1462–4.
70. Vilela EG, Ferrari M, Torres H, et al. Influence of Saccharomyces boulardii on the intestinal permeability of patients with Crohn's disease in remission. Scand J Gastroenterol 2008;43:842–8.
71. Bousvaros A, Guandalini S, Baldassano RN, et al. A randomized, double-blind trial of Lactobacillus GG versus placebo in addition to standard maintenance

therapy for children with Crohn's disease. Inflamm Bowel Dis 2005;11(9): 833–9.

72. Prantera C, Scribano ML, Falasco G, et al. Ineffectiveness of probiotics in preventing recurrence after curative resection for Crohn's disease: a randomised controlled trial with Lactobacillus GG. Gut 2002;51(3):405–9.

73. Marteau P, Lemann M, Seksik P, et al. Ineffectiveness of Lactobacillus johnsonii LA1 for prophylaxis of postoperative recurrence in Crohn's disease: a randomised, double blind, placebo controlled GETAID trial. Gut 2006;55(6):842–7.

74. Rolfe VE, Fortun PJ, Hawkey CJ, et al. Probiotics for maintenance of remission in Crohn's disease. Cochrane Database Syst Rev 2006;(4):CD004826.

75. Rahimi R, Nikfar S, Rahimi F, et al. A meta-analysis on the efficacy of probiotics for maintenance of remission and prevention of clinical and endoscopic relapse in Crohn's disease. Dig Dis Sci 2008;53(9):2524–31.

76. Shen J, Ran HZ, Yin MH, et al. Meta-analysis: the effect and adverse events of Lactobacilli versus placebo in maintenance therapy for Crohn disease. Intern Med J 2009;39(2):103–9.

77. Chermesh I, Tamir A, Reshef R, et al. Failure of Synbiotic 2000 to prevent postoperative recurrence of Crohn's disease. Dig Dis Sci 2007;52(2):385–9.

78. Doherty G, Bennett G, Patil S, et al. Interventions for prevention of post-operative recurrence of Crohn's disease. Cochrane Database Syst Rev 2009;(4):CD006873.

79. Floch MH, Walker WA, Madsen K, et al. Recommendations for probiotic use-2011 update. J Clin Gastroenterol 2011;45(Suppl):S168–71.

80. Dominguez-Bello MG, Blaser MJ, Ley RE, et al. Development of the human gastrointestinal microbiota and insights from high-throughput sequencing. Gastroenterology 2011;140(6):1713–9.

81. Borody TJ, Warren EF, Leis S, et al. Treatment of ulcerative colitis using fecal bacteriotherapy. J Clin Gastroenterol 2003;37(1):42–7.

82. Guslandi M, Giollo P, Testoni PA. A pilot trial of Saccharomyces boulardii in ulcerative colitis. Eur J Gastroenterol Hepatol 2003;15(6):697–8.

83. Kato K, Mizuno S, Umesaki Y, et al. Randomized placebo-controlled trial assessing the effect of bifidobacteria-fermented milk on active ulcerative colitis. Aliment Pharmacol Ther 2004;20(10):1133–41.

84. Tursi A, Brandimarte G, Giorgetti GM, et al. Low-dose balsalazide plus a high-potency probiotic preparation is more effective than balsalazide alone or mesalazine in the treatment of acute mild-to-moderate ulcerative colitis. Med Sci Monit 2004;10(11):PI126–31.

85. Venturi A, Gionchetti P, Rizzello F, et al. Impact on the composition of the faecal flora by a new probiotic preparation: preliminary data on maintenance treatment of patients with ulcerative colitis. Aliment Pharmacol Ther 1999;13(8):1103–8.

86. Cui HH, Chen CL, Wang JD, et al. Effects of probiotic on intestinal mucosa of patients with ulcerative colitis. World J Gastroenterol 2004;10(10):1521–5.

87. Laake KO, Line PD, Grzyb K, et al. Assessment of mucosal inflammation and blood flow in response to four weeks' intervention with probiotics in patients operated with a J-configurated ileal-pouch-anal-anastomosis (IPAA). Scand J Gastroenterol 2004;39(12):1228–35.

88. Gionchetti P, Rizzello F, Venturi A, et al. Oral bacteriotherapy as maintenance treatment in patients with chronic pouchitis: a double-blind, placebo-controlled trial. Gastroenterology 2000;119(2):305–9.

89. Malchow HA. Crohn's disease and Escherichia coli. A new approach in therapy to maintain remission of colonic Crohn's disease? J Clin Gastroenterol 1997;25(4): 653–8.

Probiotics, Prebiotics, Energy Balance, and Obesity
Mechanistic Insights and Therapeutic Implications

Federica Molinaro, MD[a,1], Elena Paschetta, MD[a,1], Maurizio Cassader, PhD[a], Roberto Gambino, PhD[a], Giovanni Musso, MD[b,*]

KEYWORDS

• Microbiota • Endotoxin • Obesity • Probiotics • Prebiotics

KEY POINTS

- Increased consumption of foods with high energy is involved in obesity development, which is a well-known risk factor for type 2 diabetes mellitus (T2DM) and cardiovascular disease.
- Several studies have demonstrated that gut microbiota can modulate host energy homeostasis and adiposity through different mechanisms: energy harvest from diet, fat storage and expenditure, incretins secretion, and systemic inflammation.
- Although experimental data suggest gut microbiota manipulation with probiotics and prebiotics can beneficially affect host adiposity and glucose metabolism, their effects are transient and diminish gradually after cessation.
- This review analyzes the potential gut microbiota-driven pathways that could represent novel target for treatment of obesity.

INTRODUCTION

Obesity-related disorders are related to energy homeostasis and inflammation; gut microbiota are involved in several host metabolic functions and may play an important role in this context through several mechanisms: increased energy harvest from the diet, regulation of host metabolism, and modulation of inflammation.

Human gut flora comprises at least 10^{14} bacteria belonging to 3 bacterial phyla: the gram-positive Firmicutes and Actinobacteria and the gram-negative Bacteroidetes.

[a] Department of Medical Sciences, Corso AM Dogliotti 14 10124, University of Turin, Italy;
[b] Department of Emergency Medicine, Gradenigo Hospital, Gradenigo Hospital, Turin, Corso Regina Margherita 8, Turin 10132, Italy
[1] Equal first author.
* Corresponding author.
E-mail address: giovanni_musso@yahoo.it

Gastroenterol Clin N Am 41 (2012) 843–854
http://dx.doi.org/10.1016/j.gtc.2012.08.009
0889-8553/12/$ – see front matter © 2012 Elsevier Inc. All rights reserved.

gastro.theclinics.com

Firmicutes is the largest bacterial phylum and comprises more than 200 genera, including *Lactobacillus, Mycoplasma, Bacillus*, and *Clostridium* species.[1] Although each subject has a specific gut microbiota, a core human gut microbiome is shared among family members despite different environments[2]; nevertheless, the microbiome dynamically changes in response to some factors, including dietary nutrients, illness, and antibiotic use.

This review discusses the interaction of gut microbiota with host metabolism and the impact of manipulating microbiota composition on the pathogenesis and the treatment of obesity.

ASSOCIATION BETWEEN GUT MICROBIOTA AND OBESITY: PATHOPHYSIOLOGICAL MECHANISMS

Several data suggest that gut microflora play a role in the regulation of host energy homeostasis (**Table 1**).

Table I
Gut microbiota modulation of host energy homeostasis: mechanisms

Mechanisms	Mediators	Metabolic Effects
Reduced intestinal transit rate	Production of SCFA , that increase Gpr41-/Gpr43-mediated PYY secretion	Increased energy harvest from the diet
Polysaccharide degradation to monosaccharides	Microbial transport proteins and enzymes	Increased CHO absobtion and portal flow
Increased glucose absorption	Increased intestinal Glut1 expression	
Increased monosaccharides portal low	Increased capillaries density in intestinal villi	
Increased de novo lipogenesis	ChREBP and SREBP-1 mediated expression of lipogenic enzyme	Increased hepatic/adipose Tg contents
Increased adipociyte uptake of circulating FFA	Increased adipose LPL activity through reduction of intestinal Fiaf secretion	
Reduced FFA oxidation	Reduced Fiaf-induced (PGC)-1α and AMPK-induced expression of mitochondrial FFA oxidative enzymes	Reduced hepatic/muscle FFA oxidation
Regulation of GLP-2 secretion	Modulation of intestinal L-cell activity	Modulation of intestinal barrier function
LPS production	LPS-TLR4-mediated induction of hepatic/adipose/macrophagical pro-inflammatory cytokines SOCS-1, SOCS-3, IL-6, TNF-α, MCP-1	Modulation of systemic/hepatic/adipose inflammation
Modulation of gut barrier integrity	Stimulation of L-cell differentiation and GLP-2 secretion	
Regulation of hepatic/adipose fatty acid composition	Increased linoleic acid conversion to c9, t11 CLA , increased hepatic and adipose contents of DHA and EPA	Modulation of tissue composition of fatty acid

Animal models suggest obesity is associated with alteration of gut microbiota: germ-free mice have less total body fat than conventionally raised mice. The colonization of germ-free mice with a normal microbiota (composed mainly of *Bacteroides* and *Clostridium* genera) results in an increase in total body fat, hepatic triglycerides, fasting plasma glucose, and insulin resistance, despite a reduced food intake.[3] Similarly, conventionalization of germ-free mice with flora from obese donors induces a greater increase in total body fat than colonization with microbiota from lean mice.[4]

Moreover, germ-free mice are protected against the Western diet–induced insulin resistance and gained less body weight and fat mass than conventionalized mice.[5]

Genetically obese leptin-deficient ob/ob mice harbour a significantly higher percentage of Firmicutes and a 50% lower percentage of Bacteroidetes compared with their wild-type littermates fed the same polysaccharide-rich diet.[6] Consistently, in the high-fat/high-sugar Western diet mice, a model of dietary obesity, the development of obesity was associated with enrichment in Firmicutes at the expense of the Bacteroidetes compared with mice receiving a low-fat/high polysaccharide diet.[7] Metagenomic analysis of the obese microbiome showed a depletion of genes involved in motility and an enrichment in genes enabling the capacity of extract energy from the diet, including glycoside hydrolases, phosphotransferases, β-fructosidase and in other transport proteins and fermentation enzymes further processing breakdown products.

Although Bifidobacterium is not a predominating phylum in the gut, it seems to play an important role in host metabolism. In mice, a high-fat diet led to a reduction in Bifidobacterium, associated with increased fat mass, insulin resistance, and inflammatory activity.[8]

Gut microbiota is also connected to metabolic disorders through the modulation of the innate immune system. Mice genetically deficient in Toll-like receptor (TLR) 5, a component of innate immune system in the gut, developed hallmark features of metabolic syndrome, including hyperlipidemia, hypertension, insulin resistance, and increased adiposity, associated with changes in the composition of the gut microbiota. Transplantation of microbiota from TLR5-deficient mice to wild-type germ-free mice conferred many features of metabolic syndrome to the recipients.[9]

Increased Energy Harvest from the Diet

Nutrient absorption and gut motility can be modulated by short chain fatty acids (SCFAs), the major end products of bacterial fermentation. SCFAs (propionate, acetate, and butyrate) represent more than 60% of energy content of carbohydrates from the diet[10] and are ligands for Gpr41 and Gpr43, 2 G protein–coupled receptors that induce intestinal secretion of peptide YY (PYY) and leptin.

Gpr41 functional deletion was related with a reduction in PYY expression, a faster intestinal transit rate, and a reduction of energy uptake from the diet.[11] Consistently, Grp43-deficient mice showed lower total body fat and improved insulin sensitivity; moreover, GPR43 inhibition was associated with higher energy expenditure accompanied by higher core body temperature and increased food intake.[12]

Collectively, these findings disclose the pivotal role for Gpr41 and Gpr43 in mediating microbiota regulation of energy harvest from the diet.

Regulation of Host Energy Storage

In conventionalized mice, microbiota promotes absorption of monosaccharides from the gut lumen.[5] Increased carbohydrate availability promotes de novo lipogenesis in the liver and the adipose tissue by stimulating carbohydrate response element binding protein–mediated and sterol response element binding protein 1–mediated transcription of genes encoding 2 rate-limiting lipogenetic enzymes: acetyl-CoA carboxylase 1 and fatty acid synthase.[13] This mechanism leads to an accumulation of triglycerides in the liver and in adipose tissue.

Fasting-induced adipose factor (Fiaf), also called angiopoietin-like protein 4, is an inhibitor of adipose lipoprotein lipase produced by enterocytes, hepatocytes, skeletal myocytes, and adipocytes in response to fasting, peroxisome proliferator-activated receptor-γ activation, and inflammatory prostaglandins, PGD_2 and PGJ_2.[14] Fiaf also modulates fatty acid oxidation in skeletal muscle and in adipocytes, increasing the nuclear transcription factor peroxisomal proliferator-activated receptor coactivator 1α, a coactivator of genes encoding key enzymes involved in mitochondrial fatty acid oxidation.[15]

Gut microbiota affect storage of circulating triglycerides into adipocytes by regulating intestinal secretion of Fiaf: conventionalization of germ-free mice suppressed intestinal expression of Fiaf in differentiated villous epithelial cells in the ileum; consistently, germ-free Fiaf-KO mice fed a high-fat/high-carbohydrate diet were not protected against diet-induced obesity.[5] Specific microbiota has different effects on expression of Fiaf: mice fed a high-fat diet supplemented with *Lactobacillus paracasei* showed increased levels of Fiaf and displayed significantly less body fat and reduced triglyceride levels. In coculture experiments, Lactobacillus also induced Fiaf gene expression.[16] These data suggest that modulation of Fiaf through manipulating gut flora could be an important therapeutic target.

Microbiota may regulate the fatty acid metabolism also by affecting adenosine AMP–AMP (AMPK) activation. AMPK stimulates fatty acid oxidative pathways in the liver and the skeletal muscle through activation of mitochondrial enzymes, such as acetyl-CoA carboxylase and carnitine palmitoyltransferase I, and reduces hepatic glycogen-synthase activity and glycogen stores, improving hepatic and muscle insulin sensitivity.[17]

Gut flora may have an inhibitory effect on AMPK-regulated fatty acid oxidation, because germ-free mice present a persistent activation of hepatic and muscle AMPK, whereas AMPK activity and related metabolic pathways were suppressed in conventionalized mice.[5]

Regulation of Chronic Low-grade Endotoxinemia and Host Inflammatory Response

Chronic activation of the immune system is linked to the development of obesity and T2DM; TLR4-activated inflammatory pathway has been specifically connected with the low-grade chronic inflammation, which characterizes obesity-related disorders.

Gram-negative microbiota may affect host metabolism through lipopolysaccharide (LPS), which binds the complex of CD14 and TLR4 at the surface of innate immune cells, activating inflammatory pathways implicated in the pathogenesis of obesity, insulin-resistance, and T2DM.[18]

Beside LPS, free fatty acid and products from dying cell can bind TLR4 and stimulate inflammatory response in cell expressing TLR4 (gut immune cells, adipocytes, endothelial cells, tissue macrophages, hepatocytes, and hepatic Kupffer and stellate cells). The hepatic Kupffer cells may have an independent role in this contest: in mice, high-fat diet promotes the activation of Kupffer cells, resulting in insulin resistance and glucose intolerance, whereas selective depletion of these cells restores hepatic insulin sensitivity and improves whole-body and hepatic fat accumulation, without affecting adipose tissue macrophages.[19,20]

Metabolic endotoxiemia is also associated with nonalcoholic steatohepatitis, through hepatic inflammasome activation: a recent study reported, in a mouse model of nonalcoholic steatohepatitis, saturated fatty acids upregulation of the inflammasome that led to sensitization to LPS-induced inflammasome activation.[21] LPS administration modifies the gut microbiota composition (reduction of *Bifidobacteria* and *Eubacteria* spp) and determines metabolic effects, such as systemic insulin resistance, increased plasma and hepatic triglyceride content, and reduction of high-density lipoprotein levels[22,23]; mice fed a high-fat diet shown the same change in microbiota, associated with a low-grade elevation in circulating LPS levels (metabolic endotoxemia).[22] Consistently, LPS receptor deletion or changes of gut microbiota composition induced by antibiotic administration prevented the metabolic alteration of a high-fat diet.[22]

Modification in gut microbiota composition results in change of metabolic endotoxiemia level: prebiotic fermentable oligofructose (OFS) administration increased the intestinal proportion of *Lactobacilli* and *Bifidobacteria* in ob/ob mice, restored normal intestinal permeability through stimulation of epithelial tight-junction proteins, and reduced systemic endotoxiemia, in association with enhanced intestinal glucagon-like peptide (GLP)-2 levels.[24]

Gut microbiota modulates the gut-derived peptide secretion, promoting L-cell differentiation in the proximal colon of rats and increasing GLP-1 secretion in response to a meal in healthy humans[2]; deletion of GLP-1 abolished the beneficial effects of prebiotics on weight gain, glucose metabolism, and inflammatory pathway activation.[25] Furthermore, gut microbiota may modulate gut barrier integrity and endotoxinemia through GLP-2, a 33-amino acid peptide with known intestinotrophic properties, which is cosecreted with GLP-1 by enteroendocrine L cells.

Ob/ob mice treated with prebiotic plus carbohydrates diet presented an increased circulating GLP-1 and GLP-2, which were associated with an altered gut flora composition (increased proportion of *Lactobacilli* and *Bifidobacteria*), restored tight junction integrity and intestinal barrier function, and lowered endotoxinemia.[24] Administration of a GLP-2 antagonist prevented these effects, which were mimicked by the administration of a GLP-2 agonist, suggesting that GLP-2 could mediate the effects of prebiotics.[24]

Microbiota, such as *Bifidobacterium* and *Lactobacillus*, may exert an anti-inflammatory effect through the synthesis of bioactive isomers of conjugated linoleic acid, which shows antidiabetic, antiatherosclerotic, hypocholesterolemic, hypotriglyceridemic, and immunomodulatory activity.[26,27]

In different mammalian models, dietary supplementation of linoleic acid plus *Bifidobacterium breve* altered the profile of polyunsaturated fatty acid composition, resulting in higher intestinal, hepatic, and adipose tissue content of c9,t11 conjugated linoleic acid; the animals also present a higher adipose tissue concentrations of eicosapentaenoic acid and docosahexaenoic acid, 2 omega-3 polynsatured fatty acids with anti-inflammatory and lipid-lowering properties.[28] These changes were associated with a reduced expression of proinflammatory cytokines, such as tumor necrosis factor α, interleukin-6, interleukin-1β, and interleukin-8, accompanied with a higher anti-inflammatory interleukin-10 secretion.

Finally, SCFAs elevation also could result in a reduction of the inflammation and an improvement of insulin sensitivity. Butyrate shows anti-inflammatory properties that could improve epithelial permeability.[29] Acetate raised plasma PYY and GLP-1 and suppressed proinflammatory cytokines.[30]

Collectively, these data suggest that endotoxinemia is involved in the pathogenesis of obesity-related diseases, is affected by dietary nutrient composition, and may be modulated by manipulation of gut microbiota composition.

The Role of Vitamin D

Vitamin D deficiency has been associated with allergic diseases development and increased body mass index.[31]

Vitamin D plays a role in immunomodulation and a decreased vitamin D uptake has been correlated with a change in fecal microbiota composition in one study,[32] although this association needs to be confirmed in larger cohorts.

Mice lacking the vitamin D receptor present chronic, low-grade inflammation in the gastrointestinal tract[33] and the absence of the vitamin D receptor results in enhanced inflammation in response to normally nonpathogenic bacterial flora.[34] Moreover, intestinal vitamin D receptor has also been shown to negatively regulate bacterial-induced intestinal nuclear factor κB activation and to attenuate response to infection, suggesting that the vitamin D may affect the impact of intestinal flora on inflammatory disorders.[35]

THE ROLE OF GUT MICROBIOTA IN HUMAN OBESITY

Obese humans show an increase in Firmicutes/Bacteroidetes ratio; dietary-induced or surgically induced weight loss results in a reduction in this ratio, with a proportion of Bacteroidetes and Firmicutes similar to that found in lean humans, irrespective of the type of diet (fat or carbohydrate restricted).[36–40]

A metagenomic analysis of 154 individuals, including monozygotic and dizygotic twins concordant for leanness or obesity, and their mothers also showed that obesity was associated with a relative depletion of Bacteroidetes and a higher proportion of Actinobacteria compared with leanness.[2] Consistently, one prospective study found that children with lower proportion of Bifidobacterium and higher levels of *Staphylococus aureus* in their infancy gained significantly more weight at 7 years.[41]

The aforementioned changes in gut microbiota composition in human obesity were not uniformly found by different investigators. Some investigators reported no differences or even lower ratios of Firmicutes to Bacteroidetes in obese human adults compared with lean controls; however, significant diet dependent reductions in a group of butyrate-producing Firmicutes were found.[38,42] Arumugam and colleagues[43] investigated the phylogenetic composition of 39 fecal samples from individuals representing 6 nationalities. They characterized 3 clusters of individual microbiotal composition, referred to as enterotypes, that were not nation specific or continent specific. They identified 3 marker molecules that correlate strongly with the host's body mass index, 2 of which are ATPase complexes, supporting the link found between energy harvest and obesity in the host and suggesting the importance of metagenomic-derived functional biomarkers over phylogenetic ones.

Changes in energy harvesting from diet is also associated with the uptake of SCFAs, end products of bacterial fermentation: in obese humans, the amount of SCFAs in fecal samples was greater than in lean subjects,[42] although the diets rich in nondigestible fibers decrease body weight and severity of diabetes[44]; these contradictory findings could be explained by the anti-inflammatory effects of butyrate.

Furthermore, another pathway has been better studied in humans: the linkage between microbiota and systemic inflammation. LPS administration induces acute inflammation and systemic insulin resistance, stimulating the systemic and adipose tissue expression of proinflammatory and insulin resistance-inducing cytokines.[45]

Consistently in healthy human subjects, total energy intake and high-fat/high-carbohydrate meals, but not fruit/fiber meals, can acutely increased plasma LPS levels, coupled with enhanced TLR4 expression.[22,46]

In summary, the different pathophysiologic factors that explain the association of microbiota with metabolic disturbances have not been studied in depth in human in comparison with animal models, although growing evidences link gut microbiota with endotoxemia and energy harvest from diet.

THERAPEUTIC TARGETS

The mechanisms connecting gut microbiota to obesity could have relevant implications for treatment.

Probiotics

Probiotics are food supplements that contain living bacteria, such as *Bifidobacteria, Lactobacilli, Streptococci*, and nonpathogenic strains of *Escherichia coli*. When administered, they confer beneficial effects to the host because of changes in the gut microbiota that are transient and diminish gradually with time after cessation.[47] Different studies suggest that probiotics influence the intestinal lumen rather than the gut-epithelium, possibly explaining the transient effect of probiotics.[48,49] This thesis was tested by Goossens and colleagues[48]: they compared the effects of consuming *Lactobacillus plantarum* on the microbial colonization of feces and biopsies from the ascending colon and rectum. Within fecal samples, the amount of *Lactobacilli* was significantly increased. The biopsies did not, however, confirm a growth of *Lactobacilli*. Recently, van Baarlen and colleagues[50] described changes in the expression of up to thousands of genes in duodenal biopsies after administration of 3 types of *Lactobacilli*. Alterations in the gut microbiota as a result of probiotics are commonly observed but evidence showing that probiotica administration directly affects inflammatory state has only recently been demonstrated in humans.[51,52] In contrast, studies on the effects of probiotics on characteristics of T2DM are mostly performed in animal models, reporting beneficial effects by various strains of *Lactobacilli* on characteristics of T2DM.[47] Both antidiabetic and anti-inflammatory effects of *Lactobacillus casei* in diet-induced obese mice were recently described.[53] In addition, diet-induced obese mice showed a reduction in body weight gain after they were supplemented with *Lactobacillus rhamnosus PL60* plus an adequate diet.[54] In the same way, Kang and colleagues[55] studied the effects of *Lactobacillus gasseri* BNR17 on diet-induced overweight rats; they found that the percent increase in body weight and fat pad mass was significantly lower in the BNR17 group. Although these animal findings are interesting, the relevance of lactobacilli supplementation for the control of adiposity is a matter of debate. To clarify the effect of Lactobacillus-containing probiotics on weight, Million and colleagues[56] performed a meta-analysis of clinical studies and experimental models. They included 17 RCTs in humans, 51 studies on farm animals, and 14 experimental models and they concluded that different Lactobacillus species are associated different effects on weight change that are host-specific. In particular, *Lactobacillus fermentum* and *Lactobacillus ingluviei* were associated with weight gain in animals; *Lactobacillus plantarum* was associated with weight loss in animals and *Lactobacillus gasseri* was associated with weight loss both in obese humans and in animals.

Prebiotics

Prebiotics (mostly oligosaccharides) are nondigestible but fermentable food ingredients that selectively stimulate the growth or activity of one or multiple gut microbes that are beneficial to their human hosts.[47] The beneficial metabolic effects of prebiotics are in part mediated by a reduction in metabolic endotoxiemia. In physiologic situations, *Bifidobacteria* are capable of lowering LPS levels.[57,58] The number of *Bifidobacteria* was inversely correlated with the development of fat mass, glucose intolerance, and LPS level.[57] High-fat diets promote the growth of LPS-producing gut microbiota and subsequently restrict the amount of *Bifidobacteria*. *Bifidobacterium* spp and *Lactobacillus* spp are sensitive to the administration of certain prebiotics.[59] Prebiotics containing OFS specifically stimulate the growth of these intestinal bacteria.[60,61] OFS administration completely restored *Bifidobacteria* spp and normalized plasma endotoxin levels, leading to improved glucose tolerance, increased satiety, and weight loss in human subjects.[8,62,63] Besides modulating endotoxemia, OFS can alter metabolism in various other manners. Cani and colleagues[64] showed that effects of OFS were mediated via a GLP1-dependent pathway. High-fat–fed diabetic mice on OFS treatment demonstrated improved glucose tolerance, diminished body weight, and decreased endogenous glucose production. Either adding the GLP-1 receptor antagonist exendin 9–39 or using GLP-1 knockout mice resulted in a complete lack of the OFS-mediated beneficial effects, thus showing the causal role of GLP-1 in this pathway in animals. Attempts to translate these findings to human subjects are ambiguous, showing that OFS tends to dose dependently decrease energy intake and increase PYY plasma concentrations,[63,65] but reported effects on satiety are conflicting.[44] Everard and colleagues[66] found that in ob/ob mice, prebiotic feeding decreased Firmicutes and increased Bacteroidetes phyla, improved glucose tolerance, increased L-cell number and associated parameters (intestinal proglucagon mRNA expression and plasma GLP-1 levels), and reduced fat-mass development, oxidative stress, and low-grade inflammation. In high-fat–fed mice, prebiotic treatment improved leptin sensitivity as well as metabolic parameters. Furthermore, OFS fermentation directly affects SFCA butyrate synthesis from extracellular acetate and lactate, implicating the therapeutic potential of prebiotics.[67] In addition, insulin-type fructance decreased the activity of the endocannabinoid system (by reducing the expression of cannabinoid receptor 1, restoring the expression of anandamide-degrading enzyme, and decreasing anandamide levels in the intestinal and adipose tissues), a phenomenon that contributes to an improvement barrier function of the gut and adipogenesis.[68] Finally, insulin-type fructan prebiotics counteract the overespression of GPR43 in the adipose tissue, which is related to a decrease rate of differentiation and a reduce adipocyte size.[69] Thus, available evidence supports the hypothesis that prebiotics can influence metabolic disturbances. The beneficial effect on clinical endpoints in metabolic disturbances remains to be demonstrated in large prospective randomized controlled trials.

SUMMARY

Increased consumption of foods with high energy is involved obesity development, which is a well-known risk factor for T2DM and cardiovascular disease.

Several studies demonstrate gut microbiota can modulate host energy homeostasis and adiposity through different mechanisms: energy harvest from diet, fat storage and expenditure, incretins secretion, and systemic inflammation.

Although experimental data suggest gut microbiota manipulation with probiotics and prebiotics can beneficially affect host adiposity and glucose metabolism, their effects are transient and diminish gradually after cessation. This review analyzes the potential gut microbiota-driven pathways that could represent novel target for treatment of obesity.

REFERENCES

1. Zoetendal EG, Vaughan EE, de Vos WM. A microbial world within us. Mol Microbiol 2006;59:1639–50.
2. Turnbaugh PJ, Hamady M, Yatsunenko T, et al. A core gut microbiome in obese and lean twins. Nature 2009;457:480–4.
3. Backhed F, Ding H, Wang T, et al. The gut microbiota as an environmental factor that regulates fat storage. Proc Natl Acad Sci U S A 2004;101:15718–23.

4. Turnbaugh PJ, Ley RE, Mahowald MA, et al. An obesity-associated gut micro-biome with increased capacity for energy harvest. Nature 2006;444:1027–31.

5. Backhed F, Manchester JK, Semenkovich CF, et al. Mechanisms underlying the resistance to diet-induced obesity in germ-free mice. Proc Natl Acad Sci U S A 2007;104:979–84.

6. Ley RE, Bäckhed F, Turnbaugh P, et al. Obesity alters gut microbial ecology. Proc Natl Acad Sci U S A 2005;102:11070–5.

7. Turnbaugh PJ, Bäckhed F, Fulton L, et al. Diet-induced obesity is linked to marked but reversible alterations in the mouse distal gut microbiome. Cell Host Microbe 2008;3:213–23.

8. Cani PD, Amar J, Iglesias MA, et al. Metabolic endotoxemia initiates obesity and insulin resistance. Diabetes 2007;56:1761–72.

9. Vijay-Kumar M, Aitken JD, Carvalho FA, et al. Metabolic syndrome and altered gut microbiota in mice lacking Toll-like receptor 5. Science 2010;328:228–31.

10. Louis P, Flint HJ. Diversity, metabolism and microbial ecology of butyrate producing bacteria from the human large intestine. FEMS Microbiol Lett 2009;294:1–8.

11. Samuel BS, Shaito A, Motoike T, et al. Effects of the gut microbiota on host adiposity are modulated by the short-chain fatty acid binding G protein-coupled receptor, Gpr41. Proc Natl Acad Sci U S A 2008;105:16767–72.

12. Bjursell M, Admyre T, Göransson M, et al. Improved glucose control and reduced body fat mass in free fatty acid receptor 2-deficient mice fed a highfat diet. Am J Physiol Endocrinol Metab 2011;300:211–20.

13. Musso G, Gambino R, Cassader M. Recent insights into hepatic lipid metabolism in non-alcoholic fatty liver disease (NAFLD). Prog Lipid Res 2009;48:1–26.

14. Dutton S, Trayhurn P. Regulation of angiopoietin-like protein 4/fasting-induced adipose factor (Angptl4/FIAF) expression in mouse white adipose tissue and 3T3-L1 adipocytes. Br J Nutr 2008;100:18–26.

15. Musso G, Gambino R, Cassander M. Interactions between gut microbiota and host metabolism predisposing to obesity and diabetes. Annu Rev Med 2011;62:361–80.

16. Aronsson L, Huang Y, Parini P, et al. Decreased fat storage by Lactobacillus para-casei is associated with increased levels of angiopoietin-like 4 protein (ANGPTL4). PLoS One 2010;5:13087.

17. Musso G, Gambino R, Cassader M. Emerging molecular targets for the treatment of nonalcoholic fatty liver disease. Annu Rev Med 2010;61:375–92.

18. Seki E, Brenner DA. TLR and adaptor molecules in liver disease: update. Hepatology 2008;48:322–35.

19. Neyrinck AM, Cani PD, Dewulf EM, et al. Critical role of Kupffer cells in the management of diet-induced diabetes and obesity. Biochem Biophys Res Commun 2009;385:351–6.

20. Huang W, Metlakunta A, Dedousis N, et al. Depletion of liver Kupffer cells prevents the development of diet-induced hepatic steatosis and insulin resistance. Diabetes 2010;59:347–57.

21. Csak T, Ganz M, Pespisa J, et al. Fatty acid and endotoxin activate inflamma-somes in mouse hepatocytes that release danger signals to stimulate immune cells. Hepatology 2011;54(1):133–44.

22. Cani PD, Bibiloni R, Knauf C, et al. Changes in gut microbiota control metabolic endotoxemia-induced inflammation in high-fat diet–induced obesity and diabetes in mice. Diabetes 2008;57:1470–81.

23. Osto M, Zini E, Franchini M, et al. Subacute endotoxemia induces adipose inflam-mation and changes in lipid and lipoprotein metabolism in cats. Endocrinology 2011;152:804–15.

24. Cani PD, Possemiers S, Van de Wiele T, et al. Changes in gut microbiota control inflammation in obese mice through a mechanism involving GLP-2-driven improvement of gut permeability. Gut 2009;58:1091–103.

25. Zhou J, Martin RJ, Tulley RT, et al. Dietary resistant starch upregulates total GLP-1 and PYY in a sustained day-long manner through fermentation in rodents. Am J Physiol Endocrinol Metab 2008;295:E1160–6.

26. Gorissen L, Raes K, Weckx S, et al. Production of conjugated linoleic acid and conjugated linolenic acid isomers by *Bifidobacterium* species. Appl Microbiol Biotechnol 2010;87:2257–66.

27. Devillard E, McIntosh FM, Paillard D, et al. Differences between human subjects in the composition of the faecal bacterial community and faecal metabolism of linoleic acid. Microbiology 2009;155(Pt 2):513–20.

28. Wall R, Ross RP, Shanahan F, et al. Metabolic activity of the enteric microbiota influences the fatty acid composition of murine and porcine liver and adipose tissues. Am J Clin Nutr 2009;89:1393–401.

29. Lewis K, Lutgendorff F, Phan V, et al. Enhanced translocation of bacteria across metabolically stressed epithelia is reduced by butyrate. Inflamm Bowel Dis 2010; 16:1138–48.

30. Freeland KR, Wolever TM. Acute effects of intravenous and rectal acetate on glucagon-like peptide-1, peptide YY, ghrelin, adiponectin and tumour necrosis factor-alpha. Br J Nutr 2010;103:460–6.

31. Parikh SJ, Edelman M, Uwaifo GI, et al. The relationship between obesity and serum 1,25-dihydroxy vitamin D concentrations in healthy adults. J Clin Endocrinol Metab 2004;89:1196–9.

32. Mai V, McCrary QM, Sinha R, et al. Associations between dietary habits and body mass index with gut microbiota composition and fecal water genotoxicity: an observational study in African American and Caucasian American volunteers. Nutr J 2009;8:49.

33. Adorini L, Penna G. Dendritic cell tolerogenicity: a key mechanism in immunomodulation by vitamin D receptor agonists. Hum Immunol 2009;70:345–52.

34. Yu S, Bruce D, Froicu M, et al. Failure of T cell homing, reduced CD4/CD8alphaalpha intraepithelial lymphocytes, and inflammation in the gut of vitamin D receptor KO mice. Proc Natl Acad Sci U S A 2008;105:20834–9.

35. Wu S, Liao AP, Xia Y, et al. Vitamin D receptor negatively regulates bacterial-stimulated NF-kappaB activity in intestine. Am J Pathol 2010;177:686–97.

36. Ley RE, Turnbaugh PJ, Klein S, et al. Microbial ecology: human gut microbes associated with obesity. Nature 2006;444:1022–3.

37. Zhang H, DiBaise JK, Zuccolo A, et al. Human gut microbiota in obesity and after gastric bypass. Proc Natl Acad Sci U S A 2009;106:2365–70.

38. Duncan SH, Lobley GE, Holtrop G, et al. Human colonic microbiota associated with diet, obesity and weight loss. Int J Obes 2008;32:1720–4.

39. Santacruz A, Marcos A, Wärnberg J, et al. Interplay between weight loss and gut microbiota composition in overweight adolescents. Obesity (Silver Spring) 2009; 17:1906–15.

40. Nadal I, Santacruz A, Marcos A, et al. Shifts in clostridia, bacteroides and immunoglobulin-coating fecal bacteria associated with weight loss in obese adolescents. Int J Obes 2009;33:758–67.

41. Kalliomaki M, Collado MC, Salminen S, et al. Early differences in fecal microbiota composition in children may predict overweight. Am J Clin Nutr 2008;87:534–8.

42. Schwiertz A, Taras D, Schäfer K, et al. Microbiota and SCFA in lean and overweight healthy subjects. Obesity (Silver Spring) 2010;18(1):190–5.

43. Arumugam M, Raes J, Pelletier E, et al. Enterotypes of the human gut microbiome. Nature 2011;473(7346):174–80 [Erratum appears in Nature 2011;474(7353):666].
44. Cani PD, Joly E, Horsmans Y, et al. Oligofructose promotes satiety in healthy human: a pilot study. Eur J Clin Nutr 2006;60:567–72.
45. Mehta N, McGillicuddy FC, Anderson PD, et al. Experimental endotoxemia induces adipose inflammation and insulin resistance in humans. Diabetes 2010;59:172–81.
46. Ghanim H, Abuaysheh S, Sia CL, et al. Increase in plasma endotoxin concentrations and the expression of Toll-like receptors and suppressor of cytokine signaling-3 in mononuclear cells after a high-fat, high-carbohydrate meal: implications for insulin resistance. Diabetes Care 2009;32:2281–7.
47. Kootte RS, Vrieze A, Holleman F, et al. The therapeutic potential of manipulating gut microbiota in obesity and type 2 diabetes mellitus. Diabetes Obes Metab 2012;14(2):112–20.
48. Goossens DA, Jonkers DM, Russel MG, et al. The effect of a probiotic drink with Lactobacillus plantarum 299v on the bacterial composition in faeces and mucosal biopsies of rectum and ascending colon. Aliment Pharmacol Ther 2006;23(2):255–63.
49. Martin FP, Wang Y, Sprenger N, et al. Probiotic modulation of symbiotic gut microbial-host metabolic interactions in a humanized microbiome mouse model. Mol Syst Biol 2008;4:157.
50. van Baarlen P, Troost F, van der Meer C, et al. Human mucosal in vivo transcriptome responses to three lactobacilli indicate how probiotics may modulate human cellular pathways. Proc Natl Acad Sci U S A 2011;108(Suppl 1):4562–9.
51. Konstantinov SR, Smidt H, de Vos WM, et al. S layer protein A of Lactobacillus acidophilus NCFM regulates immature dendritic cell and T cell functions. Proc Natl Acad Sci U S A 2008;105:19474–9.
52. van Baarlen P, Troost FJ, van HS, et al. Differential NF-kappaB pathways induction by Lactobacillus plantarum in the duodenum of healthy humans correlating with immune tolerance. Proc Natl Acad Sci U S A 2009;106:2371–6.
53. Naito E, Yoshida Y, Makino K, et al. Beneficial effect of oral administration of Lactobacillus casei strain Shirota on insulin resistance in diet-induced obesity mice. J Appl Microbiol 2011;110:650–7.
54. Lee HY, Park JH, Seok SH, et al. Human originated bacteria, Lactobacillus rhamnosus PL60, produce conjugated linoleic acid and show anti-obesity effects in diet-induced obese mice. Biochim Biophys Acta 2006;1761:736–44.
55. Kang JH, Yun SI, Park HO. Effects of Lactobacillus gasseri BNR17 on body weight and adipose tissue mass in diet-induced overweight rats. J Microbiol 2010;48:712–4.
56. Million M, Angelakis E, Paul M, et al. Comparative meta-analysis of the effect of Lactobacillus species on weight gain in humans and animals. Microb Pathog 2012;53(2):100–8.
57. Cani PD, Neyrinck AM, Fava F, et al. Selective increases of bifidobacteria in gut microflora improve high-fat-diet-induced diabetes in mice through a mechanism associated with endotoxaemia. Diabetologia 2007;50:2374–83.
58. Griffiths EA, Duffy LC, Schanbacher FL, et al. In vivo effects of bifidobacteria and lactoferrin on gut endotoxin concentration and mucosal immunity in Balb/c mice. Dig Dis Sci 2004;49:579–89.
59. Meyer D, Stasse-Wolthuis M. The bifidogenic effect of inulin and oligofructose and its consequences for gut health. Eur J Clin Nutr 2009;63(11):1277–89.

60. Silk DB, Davis A, Vulevic J, et al. Clinical trial: the effects of a trans-galactooligosaccharide prebiotic on faecal microbiota and symptoms in irritable bowel syndrome. Aliment Pharmacol Ther 2009;29(5):508–18.

61. Tuohy KM, Rouzaud GC, Bruck WM, et al. Modulation of the human gut microflora towards improved health using prebiotics—assessment of efficacy. Curr Pharm Des 2005;11(1):75–90.

62. Cani PD, Lecourt E, Dewulf EM, et al. Gut microbiota fermentation of prebiotics increases satietogenic and incretin gut peptide production with consequences for appetite sensation and glucose response after a meal. Am J Clin Nutr 2009;90(5):1236–43.

63. Parnell JA, Reimer RA. Weight loss during oligofructose supplementation is associated with decreased ghrelin and increased peptide YY in overweight and obese adults. Am J Clin Nutr 2009;89(6):1751–9.

64. Cani PD, Knauf C, Iglesias MA, et al. Improvement of glucose tolerance and hepatic insulin sensitivity by oligofructose requires a functional glucagon-like peptide 1 receptor. Diabetes 2006;55:1484–90.

65. Verhoef SP, Meyer D, Westerterp KR. Effects of oligofructose on appetite profile, glucagon-like peptide 1 and peptide YY3-36 concentrations and energy intake. Br J Nutr 2011;106:1757–62.

66. Everard A, Lazarevic V, Derrien M, et al. Responses of gut microbiota and glucose and lipid metabolism to prebiotics in genetic obese and diet-induced leptin-resistant mice. Diabetes 2011;60(11):2775–86.

67. Morrison DJ, Mackay WG, Edwards CA, et al. Butyrate production from oligofructose fermentation by the human faecal flora: what is the contribution of extracellular acetate and lactate? Br J Nutr 2006;96(3):570.

68. Muccioli GG, Naslain D, Backhed F, et al. The endocannabinoid system links gut microbiota to adipogenesis. Mol Syst Biol 2010;6:392.

69. Dewulf EM, Cani PD, Nevrinck AM, et al. Inulin-type fructans with prebiotic properties counteract GPR43 overexpression and PPARγ-related adipogenesis in the white adipose tissue of high-fat diet-fed mice. J Nutr Biochem 2011;22(8):712–22.

Nucleic Acid-based Methods to Assess the Composition and Function of the Bowel Microbiota

Blair Lawley, PhD[a], Gerald W. Tannock, PhD[a,b],*

KEYWORDS

- Bowel microbiota • Probiotic • Fecal microbiota • Microbiota compositional analysis
- Microbiota functional analysis • Nucleic acid-based analysis of microbiota

KEY POINTS

- Over evolutionary time, people have developed an equilibrium with the microbial world, which consists of cloaking the body inside and out with microorganisms that are likelier to be friends than enemies.
- Nucleic acid-based methods of analysis are widely used to determine and monitor the composition of this metaphorical cloak of microbes (microbiota). This was originally because many of the members of microbiota had not yet been cultivated in the laboratory.
- Nucleic acid-based methods also facilitate logistical planning and execution of microbiota analysis for probiotic, clinical, and nutritional trials using human subjects.

IS THERE A NEED TO KNOW ABOUT MICROBIOTA COMPOSITION IN PROBIOTIC STUDIES?

Roy Fuller, a pioneer in the probiotic field, defined a probiotic as a "live microbial feed supplement which beneficially affects the host animal by improving its intestinal microbial balance."[1] This definition infers that consumption of the probiotic preparation will alter the proportions of the various populations that comprise the microbiota. There is little evidence that this happens, apart from small increases in the abundance of the taxonomic group to which the probiotic belongs. Moreover, the effect is transient, because the probiotic bacteria are only detected in feces as long as the probiotic is consumed.[2] In other words, it is a temporary addition to the microbiota of the large bowel without displacement of resident populations. There is recent evidence that the biochemistry of the microbiota may change during probiotic consumption, but

a Department of Microbiology and Immunology, University of Otago, Post Office Box 56, 720 Cumberland Street, Dunedin, New Zealand; b Riddet Institute Centre of Research Excellence, Cnr University Avenue and Orchard Road, Massey University, PO Box 11 222, Palmerston North 4442, New Zealand
* Corresponding author. Department of Microbiology and Immunology, University of Otago, Post Office Box 56, 720 Cumberland Street, Dunedin, New Zealand.
E-mail address: gerald.tannock@otago.ac.nz

Gastroenterol Clin N Am 41 (2012) 855–868
http://dx.doi.org/10.1016/j.gtc.2012.08.010
0889-8553/12/$ – see front matter © 2012 Elsevier Inc. All rights reserved.

an impact on the immune system by consumption of probiotic bacteria seems to be the main outcome predicted.[3,4] It can be argued, therefore, that probiotic stimuli are directed at the mucosal immune system of the small bowel as the bolus of bacteria progresses from stomach to colon after consumption.

Until the situation is clarified, and the mechanisms that mediate probiotic activity are discovered, it seems wise to include analysis of the fecal or other microbiota as part of human probiotic trials. The more complete the picture that is generated, the more likely that mechanistic details will be revealed.

While probiotic bacteria are allochthonous to the bowel biome, they should have the capacity to at least survive transit through the human gut after consumption to have some efficacy. Thus detection and quantification of the probiotic strain among the myriad of autochthonous commensals of the large bowel should be accomplished (see section on Why Detect Probiotic Bacteria Using Bulk DNA?).

Human probiotic trials of appropriate statistical power are difficult and expensive to set up and run. The main outcome is usually a clinical read-out such as prevalence of eczema in a test group relative to a placebo control group. Recruits to clinical trials are not usually reluctant to provide fecal samples, and at the least, these can be archived in small aliquots for later microbiota analysis when initial results make this desirable, or additional funding becomes available.

It is recommended that temporal studies of the microbiota be performed, necessitating the collection of specimens for microbiota analysis at several time points during the study. This will provide much needed information about the stability/variability of microbiota compositions over time. A major criticism of gut microbiota research is that human studies, and most experimental animal studies, are one-off; they are never repeated with another group of people or animals. Therefore the consistency of probiotic effects and microbiota composition are not known. This is in contrast to human drug trials, in which repetition of trials in more than one country is required before the drug is approved for general use.

In summary, analysis of the microbiota should be performed because

- Probiotics may yet be shown to alter the microbial component of the bowel or other biome in a subtle yet significant way.
- Efficacy of probiotic consumption is presumably related to its presence in the bowel or other body site, and this should be demonstrated.
- More complete pictures of bowel ecology are required; human trials with probiotics provide possibilities to acquire this knowledge.

WHY USE NUCLEIC ACID-BASED TOOLS IN MICROBIOTA STUDIES?

Much of the bacteriologic information about the bowel community has been generated by the use of nucleic acid-based methodologies.[5] The phylogenetic analysis (determining the phyla, families, genera, and species through molecular sequencing data and construction of data matrices) has mostly relied on comparisons of sequences of the small ribosomal subunit RNA genes (16S rRNA gene in the case of bacteria) present in DNA extracted from feces or other samples. A large database of about 2 million 16S rRNA gene sequences is currently available and provides a cornerstone of bacterial detection and identification by molecular methods.[6]

Nucleic acid-based methods of detection have indicated that most (about 90%) bacterial cells seen microscopically in terrestrial and aquatic samples, even accounting for the possibility that some are dead, have not yet been cultured in the laboratory.[7] This observation was totally unexpected in relation to traditional experiences in medical bacteriology and has been called the great plate count anomaly.

Operational taxonomic units (OTU, molecular species) never encountered in culture-based bacteriology but detectable by nucleic acid-based methods have revealed a vast, new bacterial world for investigation.

The situation with human feces is not dire, since at least 50% of the cells seen in samples can be cultivated. Additionally, representatives of most of the metabolic types of bacteria in the human colon have been cultured.[8] It is still convenient, however, to use nucleic acid-based methods to determine the composition and potential or real-time functioning of bowel communities. This is because of the diversity of bacterial types present in the bowel of people and the somewhat idiosyncratic nature of individual microbiota. Extraction of nucleic acids from feces, bowel digesta, or mucosal biopsies is now a standard procedure and is logistically much simpler than the preparation of a spectrum of selective media and anaerobic protocols that are required for culture-based investigations. Moreover, culture-based analysis requires the processing of the samples soon after collection, whereas materials for nucleic acid-based analysis can be frozen after collection and stored at low temperature (dry ice) during transport to the laboratory and while awaiting analysis. DNA, when stored at very low temperature ($-80°C$), provides a useful archive of microbial genomes that might be used in the future when advanced methodologies may increase the amount of information that can be gleaned from bulk DNA.

The starting point for nucleic acid-based analysis is the extraction of DNA or RNA directly from the fecal or other sample of interest, avoiding the need to cultivate any members of the community. A critical step in the procedure is the lysis of microbial cells to release the nucleic acids, because accurate representation of all of the microbial types in the sample is required. Although chemical methods have been used, mechanical disruption of the cells (bead-beating) is considered preferential, because even gram-positive bacterial cells, often resilient to other methods, will be lysed.

The 16S rRNA gene sequence of bacteria has become the basis of bacterial phylogeny, because it contains regions of nucleotide base sequence that are highly conserved across the bacterial world.[9] These conserved regions are interspersed with variable regions (V regions) that contain the signatures of phylogenetic groups even to species level. Therefore sequences of V regions of 16S rRNA genes are the basis of phylogenetic methods, as will be reinforced in subsequent sections of this article.

It is important to remember, however, that bulk DNA has come from any cells that were present in the sample at the time of collection. The nucleic acids may have come from resident, living, metabolizing cells, or resident, living but relatively quiescent cells or spores, from dead bacteria, or living bacteria adventitiously present at the time of collection. Detection of a particular DNA sequence in a single sample does not equate to evidence of residence of the organism in the ecosystem. Collection and analysis of samples over time are necessary to provide this evidence.

The capacity to sequence and assemble genomic information from fragments of DNA (metagenomics) or mRNA (transcriptomics) has extended the use of nucleic acids in researching the potential and actual metabolic capacity of the microbiota. These exciting approaches will be outlined in other sections of this article.

In summary, nucleic acid-based analysis of fecal or other samples from people is useful because

- It enables descriptions to be made of the phylogenetic composition of the microbiota including its yet to be cultivated members.
- It has logistical advantages with respect to transport and storage of samples.
- It enables the genetic potential of the microbiota to be determined (metagenomics).
- It enables the expression of genes at a point in time to be revealed (transcriptomics).

WHY DETECT PROBIOTIC BACTERIA USING BULK DNA?

By current definition, probiotics are live microorganisms, which when administered in adequate amounts confer a health benefit on the host.[10] Most probiotics are administered as dietary supplements either in milk-based foods or as tablets or capsules. The detection of the probiotic bacteria in fecal or other samples is not routine in efficacy trials with people. However, inclusion of an assay to detect the presence or absence of the probiotic during the progress of the trial seems a wise step, since any absence of efficacy could be due to the inability of the probiotic to survive transit through the gastrointestinal tract. Even when probiotic efficacy has been established, a mechanistic explanation is often lacking. Hence the more detailed microbiological data available that can be interrogated statistically, the better.

A study demonstrating the differential effect of 2 probiotics in the prevention of eczema and atopy provides a case in point.[11] The aim of the study was to determine whether probiotic administration in early life could prevent the development of eczema and atopy at 2 years of age. A double-blind, randomized placebo-controlled trial of infants at risk of allergic disease was performed. Pregnant women were randomized to take *Lactobacillus rhamnosus* HN001, *Bifidobacterium animalis* subspecies *lactis* HN019, or placebo, daily from 35 weeks gestation until 6 months if breast-feeding, and their infants were randomized to receive the same treatment from birth to 2 years. Four hundred and seventy-four infants were included in the study. The infants' cumulative prevalence of eczema and point prevalence of atopy (skin prick tests to common allergens) were assessed at 2 years. Infants receiving *L. rhamnosus* probiotic had a significantly reduced risk of eczema (hazard ratio [HR] 0.51, 95% confidence interval [CI] 0.30–0.85, $P = .01$) compared with placebo, but this was not the case for the *B. animalis* subspecies *lactis* group (HR 0.90, CI 0.58–1.41).

Why was one probiotic effective but the other not? One possible explanation concerned the markedly different rates of detection of the probiotics in the stools of the infants during the trial. A DNA-based technique (polymerase chain reaction [PCR] coupled with an electrophoretic detection method; see section on Electrophoretic Methods to Screen Microbiota Compositions) showed that *B. animalis* subspecies *lactis* prevalence in fecal samples increased progressively over the course of the study, from 22.6% of infants at 3 months to 53.1% of infants at 24 months. In contrast, detection of *L. rhamnosus* was greatest at 3 months, at 71.5% of babies, and slightly lower at 24 months, at 62.3% among infants administered this probiotic. Therefore, the efficacious probiotic (*L. rhamnosus*) was commonly present in the bowel of the infants from an early age, whereas the ineffective probiotic did not seem to transit the gut in about half of the infants.

An indication of the numbers of probiotic bacteria in fecal samples could give additional interpretative data in trials with people. However, it must be kept in mind that absolute guarantees of specificity (quantifying only a specific strain—the probiotic— in samples collected from nature) require a cautionary interpretation. Limited numbers of strains of the probiotic species are usually available, either in laboratory collections or in the form of genome sequences. Therefore, validation of specificity of the nucleic acid-based method is subject to relatively limited knowledge when the study was designed and performed.

In summary, detection of probiotic strains in feces by DNA-based assays

- Demonstrates that the probiotic bacteria have at least survived transit through the gut (although viability cannot be demonstrated)
- May aid in the interpretation of efficacy outcomes in trials of probiotics with people

ELECTROPHORETIC METHODS TO SCREEN MICROBIOTA COMPOSITIONS

A relatively simple, semiquantitative screening method to compare the bacterial compositions of multiple samples is provided by PCR coupled with gradient gel electrophoresis.[12] Either a chemical gradient (denaturing gradient gel electrophoresis, DGGE) or temperature gradient (temporal temperature gel electrophoresis, TTGE) is used. A V region of bacterial 16S rRNA genes is amplified from bulk DNA from samples using PCR. The PCR primers anneal with conserved sequences that span the selected V region. One of the primers has a GC-rich 5′ end (GC clamp) to prevent complete denaturation of the amplified DNA fragments during gel electrophoresis. The amplified DNA theoretically contains 16S rRNA gene sequences from all of the members of the microbiota in the sample. All of the amplified fragments are of the same size. A polyacrylamide gel is used to separate the fragments of 16S rRNA gene sequences that originated in different kinds of bacteria. The double-stranded fragments of DNA migrate in an electrical current through the polyacrylamide gel until they reach chemical or thermal conditions that represent their melting point (separation of polynucleotide strands). The migration rate of the partially denatured fragments (remember the GC clamp) is slowed. Because of the variation in the 16S rRNA gene sequences between phylogenetic groups, the DNA fragments from different kinds of bacteria have different melting points and hence show different migrations in the gel. Profiles of microbiota composition can be generated once the electrophoretic gel has been stained to reveal bands of DNA. Images of these profiles can be compared using computer software.

For example, differential clustering of bowel biopsy-associated bacteria of specimens collected in Mexico and Canada was demonstrated using PCR-TTGE.[13] Bacterial collections associated with bowel biopsies, aspirates of residual fluid after pre-endoscopy cleansing, and feces from inflammatory bowel diseases (IBD) patients and healthy subjects in Edmonton, Canada, and Mexico City, Mexico, were investigated. PCR-TTGE produced profiles of the bacterial collections whose similarities were compared. Similarity analysis showed that the profiles did not cluster according to disease status, but the Canadian and Mexican profiles could be differentiated by this method. Comparison of biopsy, aspirate, and fecal samples obtained from the same subject showed that, on average, the profiles were highly similar. Therefore, biopsy-associated bacteria are likely to represent, at least in part, contaminants from the fluid, which resembles a fecal solution, that pools in the bowel after cleansing before endoscopy.

Individual fragments of DNA can be cut from electrophoretic gels, further amplified and cloned in a surrogate host (*Escherichia coli*), then sequenced.[14] The sequence can be compared with those in 16S rRNA gene databanks to obtain identification of the bacterium from which the sequence originated. PCR primers specific for particular groups of bacteria (for example lactic acid bacteria), rather than universal primers used to detect all bacteria, can be designed.[15] These primers produce simpler profiles that can be useful in the detection of bacterial species commonly used as probiotics.

In summary, electrophoretic methods such as DGGE and TTGE

- Provide comparative snapshots of microbiota
- Can detect, using appropriate PCR primer design, specific bacterial groups within the microbiota

FLUORESCENT PROBES

DNA probes (oligonucleotides) can be designed using information in DNA databases. They specifically target (anneal to) V region sequences in bacterial 16S rRNA or 23S rRNA (large ribosomal subunit). The probes are synthesized with a 5′ label consisting of a fluorescent dye. The probes bind to target sequences within bacterial cells, enabling the bacteria to be detected and quantified. This method is referred to as 'fluorescence in situ hybridization' (FISH). Bacterial cells within which hybridization with a probe has occurred fluoresce when stimulated with appropriate wavelengths of light and hence can be detected and counted by epifluorescence microscopy or fluorescence-activated flow cytometry (FC).[16] Permeabilization of the bacterial cells in samples is required to standardize intracellular access of DNA probes to their targets. Other technical considerations include

- The physiologic state of the bacterial cells, because the number of ribosomes per bacterial cell is greater the higher the metabolic activity; bacterial cells in a quiescent state will have weak fluorescence and may not be detected
- Hybridization stringency determined by temperature, salt and formamide concentrations
- The need to check the specificity of probes by reference to databanks; new sequences are constantly added.

Clostridium difficile infection (CDI) is the most common identifiable cause of diarrhea in hospitalized patients. Current therapies rely on the administration of metronidazole or vancomycin, which reduce vegetative populations of *C. difficile* in the bowel. Recurrence of the disease when treatment with these antibiotics ceases indicates that metronidazole and vancomycin affect not only *C. difficile* but also commensal populations that normally mediate competitive exclusion. Fidaxomicin is a new antibiotic that inhibits *C. difficile*. PCR-TTGE and FISH/FC were used in a study of 23 patients with mild-to-moderate CDI to determine the different impacts of vancomycin and fidaxomicin on the composition of the fecal microbiota.[17] Multidimensional scaling (production of a similarity matrix for pair-wise comparisons of TTGE profiles) indicated that the microbiota of fidaxomicin-treated patients was different from that of vancomycin-treated subjects. FISH/FC analysis showed that clostridial cluster XIVa and clostridial cluster IV populations increased during and after the fidaxomicin treatment period. Clostridial cluster XIVa populations were similar to those in the feces of healthy control subjects by day 10. In contrast, vancomycin treatment greatly reduced the proportions of the clostridial clusters, and also of bifidobacteria, by day 10 of treatment. Outgrowth of enterobacteria coincided with the decrease in other phylogenetic groups. Overall, vancomycin treatment was characterized by a decrease in the proportions of obligately anaerobic bacteria that normally populate the human colon, and an outgrowth of facultatively anaerobic and microaerobic bacterial groups during the treatment period. These findings help to explain the substantially reduced rates of relapse following treatment of CDI with fidaxomicin in recent clinical trials; fidaxomicin is sparing of the bowel commensals that normally regulate *C. difficile* population sizes in the gut.

In summary, FISH/FC

- Detects and quantifies specific groups of bacteria (even to species level) in fecal and other samples
- Can be used to screen the microbiota for major alterations in composition
- Quantifies bacterial cells rather than DNA sequences and so is more easily related to traditional bacteriologic methods

MEASURING ABUNDANCE OF BACTERIAL GROUPS BY QUANTITATIVE PCR

PCR is a powerful tool for the detection of nucleic acid targets (both phylogenetic and functional). The utility of PCR can be further enhanced when it is used not only to detect a target but also to measure abundance of that target.

PCR requires the following components: a target DNA molecule (template), primers (short single-stranded oligonucleotides), a thermostable DNA polymerase, and free nucleotides (dNTPs). The reaction begins with a denaturation phase in which the template DNA strands are separated. The primers then bind, 1 to each strand, bracketing a region of DNA that may range from tens to thousands of nucleotides (the annealing phase). Using the primers as starting points, the DNA polymerase extends complementary DNA strands by incorporating dNTPs in a 5′ to 3′ direction (the extension phase). Thus the region of interest is effectively duplicated. The whole process is repeated multiple times (usually 30–40 cycles), and the quantity of target DNA doubles with each cycle.

PCR becomes quantitative when the amplified fragments are detected in real time after each cycle. To do this, most methods rely on either incorporation of a fluorescent dye or release of a fluorescent signal from a DNA-binding probe. The signal is recorded by a sensitive camera or spectrophotometer.[18] When the starting quantity of a template is high, a signal will be detected at an early cycle, while if the initial quantity of a template is low, many cycles of PCR will be required before a signal can be observed. Absolute quantitation of a target sequence is achieved when a standard curve, prepared using known quantities of template, is generated and subsequently used to quantify unknown samples.

The specificity of the reaction can be modified through careful design of the primer sequences. Primers can be designed to target individual species, genera, families, phyla, or kingdoms. Thus primer combinations may be used to quantify as broad or narrow a microbial group as is required.[19]

Quantitative PCR (qPCR) can be time consuming and technically demanding (especially primer design) and is a relatively low-throughput technique. As such, it is often used in conjunction with other methods as a confirmatory tool or a means of quantifying specific targets or groups within a microbiota.

Hartman and colleagues[20] assayed bacterial populations in the small bowel of patients who had undergone small bowel transplant. qPCR was used to measure changes in the relative proportions of 4 bacterial groups (*Enterobacteriales, Lactobacillales, Clostridiales,* and *Bacteroidales*) in addition to total bacterial load. Post-transplant samples, before ileostomy closure, were considered to be abnormal, because they were dominated by facultative anaerobes or microaerobic bacteria (*Enterobacteriales* and *Lactobacillales*). After closure of the ileostomy, the relative proportion of strict anaerobes increased, thus returning the community to what was considered a more normal state. The authors concluded that the population shift was due to oxygen entering the small bowel through the ileostomy. This study implies flexibility within the ileal microbiota, whereby ecological factors can drive population change over relatively short time frames.

In summary, qPCR

- Can be adapted to quantify narrow (species) to broad range (phyla) targets within a microbiota
- Is often used as an adjunct, confirmatory tool to support other quantitative or semiquantitative methodologies

DNA CHIPS TO SCREEN MICROBIOTA COMPOSITIONS

Microarrays have been a mainstay of gene expression studies for many years; however, the technology is also amenable to phylogenetic analyses of microbial communities. The first phylogenetic analysis arrays were used to identify nitrifying bacteria from environmental samples,[21] but the approach has subsequently been adapted and used, especially in Europe, to study the human microbiota.

Arrays are created by attaching specific nucleotide probes to a solid substrate, often a glass slide. Many thousands of probes are bound to the surface in a grid pattern. The design of the probes is critical to the specificity and quantitative nature of the assay, as cross-hybridization may lead to overestimation of species abundance.

DNA is extracted from the sample to be tested, and the 16S rRNA gene is amplified using universal primers. The forward primer is modified to incorporate a T7 promoter sequence upstream of the 16S rRNA-specific region. Following the amplification step, RNA copies of the amplicons are generated via the T7 promoter sequence. Modified uridine-5'-triphosphate (UTP) molecules are included for the in vitro transcription step and post-transcription labeling performed with a fluorescent molecule. The labeled RNA molecules are then hybridized to the array. Hybridization of fluorescent target molecules to the array probes is detected with a highly sensitive scanner, and platform-specific software is used to normalize signals, generate quantitative data, and identify which phylogenetic targets are present in the sample.

The Human Intestinal Tract Chip (HITChip) was developed using a curated database of 16S rRNA gene sequences retrieved from the human bowel and generated probes to the V1 and V6 regions.[22] Probes (4809 in total) were designed to target 1140 different human microbiota phylotypes at various phylogenetic levels ranging from order (10% of probes) to genus (20% of probes) to species (60% of probes). The assay was validated by identifying 40 clones from human microbiota clone libraries and was shown to be reproducible across samples. The array was also shown to be capable of relative quantification by testing artificial mixtures of phylotypes, with an estimated detection limit of 0.1% abundance. The authors subsequently demonstrated the quantitative potential of the array by reporting good correlation of data derived from HITChip experiments with data from FISH and qPCR studies. Finally the HITChip platform was used to analyze the temporal dynamics of the microbiota of young and elderly adults over a 2-month period. The results showed that the microbiota of an individual was relatively stable over a short period of time, while subjects clustered according to age, suggesting a definable change in microbiota with age.

In summary, phylogenetic microarrays, although of relatively limited usage so far:

- Provide rapid, relatively low-cost phylogenetic analysis of defined microbial communities
- Can target down to species level and be modified to incorporate new species as they are discovered
- Provide quantitative estimates of microbial groups

PHYLOGENETIC ANALYSIS—DETAILED MICROBIOTA COMPOSITION

Improved DNA sequencing technologies allow phylogenetic analysis of microbiota using numbers of samples and depth of coverage not previously considered feasible. Next-generation or high-throughput sequencing (HTS) platforms generate thousands of sequences across hundreds of samples in a single analytical run.[23] To date, most microbiota studies have utilized 1 of 2 platforms (Roche/454 [454 Life Sciences, Branford, CT, USA] pyrosequencing or Illumina bridge amplification [Illumina Inc, San Diego, CA, USA] sequencing). Early studies focused on sequencing PCR amplicons from short regions of the 16S rRNA gene.[24] Genome sequencing of hundreds of bacterial strains isolated from human feces has led to shotgun sequencing of microbiota DNA and phylogenetic inference from databases containing these whole genome sequences.[25]

Phylogenetic analysis of community composition frequently requires amplification of all or part of the 16S rRNA gene. An informed choice of primers is a critical step. Poorly designed primers can bias amplification reactions in favor of, or against, entire bacterial groups. An example is the study by Palmer and colleagues,[26] in which universal bacterial primers were used to analyze human infant microbiota from birth through the first year of life. This study concluded that bifidobacteria were a minor and likely unimportant phylogenetic group (contrary to most other studies). In retrospect, it is likely that the forward amplification primer, which contained several mismatches to bifidobacterial 16S rRNA gene sequences, led to an under-representation of this genus.

HTS chemistry is capable of only short sequence reads (100–500 bases); thus analysis of a short highly informative hypervariable region is the best choice (the V3 and V4 regions of 16S rRNA genes are commonly used).[27] 16S rRNA gene primers are appended, at the 5′ end, with adapter sequences (specific for each platform) and a short unique barcode sequence (usually 8–12 bases). Individual barcoded primer sets are then used to amplify DNA extracted from each sample. Amplicons from multiple samples are then pooled in equimolar amounts, and the entire primer pool is sequenced on the platform of choice. Several detailed bioinformatics pipelines are available for down-stream data analysis, with most following a similar format: sequence quality control, splitting of multiplexed (barcoded) sequences into individual sample pools, alignment of sequences, choice of operational taxonomic units (OTUs, phylotypes, molecular species) at a chosen level of specificity, selection of representative sequences from each OTU, discernment of taxonomic identity of each OTU, use of OTU tables to generate diversity (alfa, within sample, and beta, between sample), and other metadata-driven analyses.[6,28,29]

The value of amplicon sequencing can be seen in a study aimed at describing a putative core fecal microbiota in lean and obese twins.[30] The authors characterized the fecal microbiota of adult female monozygotic (n = 31) and dizygotic (n = 23) twin pairs, concordant for leanness or obesity, and their mothers (n = 46), and looked for effects of genotype, environmental exposure, and host adiposity on the composition of the fecal microbiota. Analysis of nearly 2 million partial 16S rRNA gene sequences revealed a distinct decrease in diversity of microbiota from obese subjects along with a shift at the phylum level toward a microbiota with lower *Bacteroidetes* and higher *Actinobacteria* proportions. Two samples (separated by approximately 57 days) were collected from each participant, and sequence analysis showed that microbiota was more similar within an individual over time than between individuals. Also, families had more similar microbiota than unrelated individuals; however, there was no difference in the degree of similarity between monozygotic and dizygotic twins. Evidence of a phylogenetic core within the fecal microbiota was not obtained since no OTU was present at greater than 0.5% abundance within any sample, and no OTU was present in all samples. In addition to the phylogenetic analysis, the authors performed a metagenomic screen (see section on Metagenomics -Determining Microbiota Biochemical Capacity) using a subset of subjects. This analysis of the fecal microbiota showed the presence of a functional core (at the gene level) rather than a phylogenetic core.

In summary, phylogenetic analysis

- Is useful in describing and comparing microbiota across different sampling groups
- Enables the in-depth study of large numbers of microbiota
- Will detect previously unidentified microbiota members
- Provides a relative quantification (abundance) of microbiota members

METAGENOMICS—DETERMINING MICROBIOTA BIOCHEMICAL CAPACITY

The term metagenomics (comparisons of genomes that are similar but not identical) covers the process in which the shotgun sequencing of bulk DNA extracted from an entire microbiota is performed with the aim of identifying the genetic characteristics and therefore the biochemical potential of its members. Initial metagenomic studies utilized cloning vectors capable of incorporating large DNA fragments.[31] These large fragments were then sequenced using Sanger sequencing chemistry. HTS platforms have removed the need for the cloning step and instead allow direct sequencing of fragmented bulk DNA. The success of metagenomic studies relies heavily on well-curated and annotated databases of whole genomes and functional genes such as are available through Genbank (The US National Institute of Health Genetic Sequence Database),[32] Kyoto encyclopedia of genes and genomes,[33] and JGI (The US Department of Energy Joint Genome Institute).[34]

A basic protocol for metagenome library preparation would include: DNA extraction, fragmentation of genomic DNA, blunt-ending of DNA fragments, A-tailing, sequence adapter ligation, size selection, and library preamplification. As for amplicon sequencing, many samples can be barcoded and analyzed in the same sequence run. The 2 main platforms are the Roche/454-FLX (titanium chemistry) and the Illumina GAII or HiSeq instruments. The advantage of the FLX is its long read length (good for poorly defined communities), while the advantage of the Illumina instruments is the large number of sequences they provide (ideal for better-defined communities). As for all sequence-based approaches, downstream bioinformatics pipelines are critical for data analysis. Short metagenomics reads are assembled into longer contiguous sequences (contigs, as per standard genome sequencing); then the assembled contigs are compared with databases of annotated genes to infer both putative function, and, if small ribosomal subunit genes are encountered, phylogenetic affiliation of the sequence.[35,36]

A recent example of metagenome sequencing of the human fecal microbiota is provided by the study of Qin and colleagues.[37] Metagenome sequences from 124 Europeans were obtained and 3.3 million nonredundant microbial genes were detected. The microbiota gene catalog was mapped to 650 bacterial and archaeal genomes, and to protein databases, providing both functional and phylogenetic information.

The authors estimated that the entire cohort contained about 1150 bacterial species with about 160 species associated with each individual. Fifty-seven species were common to more than 90% of individuals. Many species were present at very low abundance. These results supported the concept of a finite and ultimately definable fecal microbiota.

By clustering genes into functional families, a common gene set that was conserved across all subjects was detected and described as a minimal human gut metagenome. This core metagenome includes functions such as use of complex polysaccharides and synthesis of essential amino acids, vitamins, and short-chain fatty acids. In addition, some functional gene families were common to all species and hence might be described as a minimal gut bacterial genome. This included a range of housekeeping functions and a large number of rare genes with unknown function, possibly necessary for life in the human bowel.

In summary, metagenomic analysis

- Defines the functional repertoire of a microbiota
- Can be applied to large numbers of subjects with good depth per sample

METATRANSCRIPTOMICS—MICROBIOTA BIOCHEMICAL PATHWAYS IN ACTION

The detection of a species or functional gene in bulk DNA does not necessarily mean that the species or gene is active at the time of sampling. Gene expression, in general, is tightly regulated according to need under prevailing environmental conditions. While a gene catalog may be maintained within a microbiota over long periods of time, many of the genes will be switched on by microbiota members only under specific conditions.

Metatranscriptomics is a term that describes the analysis of the active gene set by sequencing mRNA molecules (gene transcripts) extracted from the microbiota.[38] This identifies the subset of a metagenome responsible for performing particular functions (eg, growth using a specific substrate present in the diet). Analysis of a metatranscriptome starts with careful definition of the ecological conditions under investigation, and consideration of the timing of sample collection (changes in gene expression may be linked closely, on a temporal scale, with environmental change). Once samples have been collected, RNA must be extracted as soon as possible, or samples should be stored in a solution that will maintain the integrity of short-lived mRNA species. The majority of RNA (up to 90%) in a bacterial cell will be ribosomal RNA.[39] This will not provide information about how the microbiota is responding biochemically to change. Therefore, rRNA is depleted from the total RNA pool by hybridizing a collection of probes that bind to rRNA of many microbial species. The probes are then selectively removed using a magnet and probe-attached magnetic beads, carrying much of the rRNA with them. The remaining RNA is now enriched with mRNA. Quantities required for direct sequencing of mRNA are sometimes higher than those obtainable from a sample and may need to be amplified. Finally, the mRNA transcripts are converted to cDNA using reverse transcription. Shotgun HTS is performed on the cDNA. Bioinformatic analysis of sequence data from a metatranscriptomic study is essentially the same as described for metagenomics. Basically, assembled open reading frames are mapped to genomic scaffolds and databases of functional protein sequences, enabling identification of overexpressed or underexpressed genes within a microbiota. The extent of the analysis may sometimes be limited by large numbers of bacterial genes that are currently annotated as hypothetical. Nevertheless, as the understanding of microbial physiology improves, so will the outcomes of metagenomic and metatranscriptomic studies.

McNulty and colleagues[3] showed the value of metatranscriptomics in their study of the impact of a probiotic on fecal microbiota. The fecal microbiota of healthy human monozygotic twin pairs was assessed before, during, and after consumption of a fermented milk product. Microbiota composition (16S rRNA gene analysis) and genetic potential (metagenomic analysis) were not altered by administration of the probiotic. Metatranscriptional analysis, however, showed changes during the period of probiotic consumption. These changes included an increase in expression of genes involved in plant polysaccharide metabolism, amino acid metabolism, and metabolism of cofactors and vitamins. While some of the upregulated transcripts could be mapped to the genomes of probiotic strains, it was thought that the presence of these bacteria led to modulation of the transcriptional activity of the resident microbiota.

In summary, metatranscriptomic analysis

- Can define the functional response of a microbiota to environmental change
- May detect rapid functional responses by the microbiota that may not involve changes in microbiota composition
- Can be applied to large numbers of subjects at good sampling depth

PUTTING IT ALL TOGETHER—MULTIVALENT ANALYSIS AT A PRACTICAL LEVEL

The methods described in this article range from the relatively simple (PCR) to the technically sophisticated (metatranscriptomics). Not all are accessible to the majority of laboratories, but a core of validated (used in more than 1 study) tools is readily available to most researchers. Reliance on a single methodology per human study is not recommended. Generally, a study could commence with a screening of samples to determine whether it will be worthwhile expending further time and money on an in-depth analysis. PCR-DGGE (TTGE) or FISH/FC are cost-effective choices for this purpose. Detailed phylogenetic investigation of the microbiota can be achieved by HTS of 16S rRNA genes that is now affordable for most laboratories. Validation of the abundances—generated by HTS—of bacterial groups of interest can be achieved by qPCR.

An example of this comprehensive approach is provided by a study of the microbiota of ileo–anal pouches.[40] Chronic pouchitis is an important long-term complication following ileal pouch–anal anastomosis for ulcerative colitis. Antibiotic administration reduces symptoms of pouchitis, indicating that bacteria have a role in pathogenesis.[41]

Fecal microbiotas of 17 patients with normal pouches (NP), 17 patients with pouchitis (CP; using samples collected from each patient when antibiotic-treated [CP-on, asymptomatic] and when untreated [CP-off, symptomatic]), and 14 familial adenomatous polyposis (FAP) patients were analyzed. An initial screen of the pouch microbiota by FISH/FC analysis revealed an expanded phylogenetic gap (comprised of bacteria that did not react with any of the commonly used FISH probes) in NP and CP-off patients relative to FAP. Antibiotic treatment reduced the gap in CP feces. Phylogenetic analysis of 16S rRNA gene sequences showed that the phylogenetic gap of CP-off patients was due to outgrowth of members of the bacterial families *Caulobacteriaceae, Sphingomonadaceae, Comamonadaceae, Peptostreptococcaceae*, and *Clostridiaceae*. The phylogenetic gap of NP stool was enriched by *Ruminococcaceae* and *Bifidobacteriaceae*. CP fecal microbiotas had reduced diversity relative to NP and FAP feces due largely to a reduction in *Lachnospiraceae/Insertae Sedis* XIV/clostridial cluster IV groups.

There was a greater diversity of phylotypes of *Clostridiaceae* in CP-off subjects. *Clostridium perfringens* was commonly associated with pouch microbiotas, but qPCR revealed that the abundance of *C perfringens* in fecal samples differed between CP-off and FAP groups, but not between CP-off and NP feces.

It was concluded that bacterial groups within the expanded phylogenetic gap of pouch patients might have roles in the pathogenesis of pouchitis. Further research concerning the physiology of cultured members of these bacterial groups would be necessary to explain their specific roles. Members of the *Lachnospiraceae, Incertae Sedis* XIV, and clostridial cluster IV could be useful biomarkers of pouch health.

In summary, a multivalent analytical approach encompasses

- A screening method, which may be semiquantitative or quantitative
- An in-depth, comparative phylogenetic analysis of microbiota composition
- Quantification, commonly by qPCR, of particular bacterial groups targeted on the basis of screening or phylogenetic analysis

REFERENCES

1. Fuller R. Probiotics in man and animals. J Appl Bacteriol 1989;66:365–78.
2. Tannock GW, Munro K, Harmsen HJ, et al. Analysis of the fecal microflora of human subjects consuming a probiotic product containing *Lactobacillus rhamnosus* DR20. Appl Environ Microbiol 2000;66:2578–88.
3. McNulty NP, Yatsunenko T, Hsiao A, et al. The impact of a consortium of fermented milk strains on the gut microbiome of gnotobiotic mice and monozygotic twins. Sci Transl Med 2011;3:106ra106.

4. Shanahan F. Molecular mechanisms of probiotic action: it's all in the strains! Gut 2011;60:1026–7.
5. Zoetendal EG, Heilig HG, Klaassens ES, et al. Isolation of DNA from bacterial samples of the human gastrointestinal tract. Nat Protoc 2006;1:870–3.
6. Cole JR, Wang Q, Cardenas E, et al. The ribosomal database project: improved alignments and new tools for rRNA analysis. Nucleic Acids Res 2009;37:D141–5.
7. Handelsman J. Metagenomics: application of genomics to uncultured microorganisms. Microbiol Mol Biol Rev 2004;68:669–85.
8. Goodman AL, Kallstrom G, Faith JJ, et al. Extensive personal human gut microbiota culture collections characterized and manipulated in gnotobiotic mice. Proc Natl Acad Sci U S A 2011;108:6252–7.
9. Woese CR. Bacterial evolution. Microbiol Rev 1987;51:221–71.
10. FAO/WHO. Joint FAO/WHO working group on drafting guidelines for the evaluation of probiotics in food. London: Joint Food and Agriculture Organization of the United Nations and World Health Organization Working Group; 2002.
11. Wickens K, Black PN, Stanley TV, et al. A differential effect of 2 probiotics in the prevention of eczema and atopy: a double-blind, randomized, placebo-controlled trial. J Allergy Clin Immunol 2008;122:788–94.
12. Muyzer G, Smalla K. Application of denaturing gradient gel electrophoresis (DGGE) and temperature gradient gel electrophoresis (TGGE) in microbial ecology. Antonie Van Leeuwenhoek 1998;73:127–41.
13. Bibiloni R, Tandon P, Vargas-Voracka F, et al. Differential clustering of bowel biopsy-associated bacterial profiles of specimens collected in Mexico and Canada: what do these profiles represent? J Med Microbiol 2008;57:111–7.
14. Snart J, Bibiloni R, Grayson T, et al. Supplementation of the diet with high-viscosity beta-glucan results in enrichment for lactobacilli in the rat cecum. Appl Environ Microbiol 2006;72:1925–31.
15. Walter J, Hertel C, Tannock GW, et al. Detection of *Lactobacillus, Pediococcus, Leuconostoc,* and *Weissella* species in human feces by using group-specific PCR primers and denaturing gradient gel electrophoresis. Appl Environ Microbiol 2001;67:2578–85.
16. Lay C, Rigottier-Gois L, Holmstrom K, et al. Colonic microbiota signatures across five northern European countries. Appl Environ Microbiol 2005;71:4153–5.
17. Tannock GW, Munro K, Taylor C, et al. A new macrocyclic antibiotic, fidaxomicin (OPT-80), causes less alteration to the bowel microbiota of *Clostridium difficile*-infected patients than does vancomycin. Microbiology 2010;156:3354–9.
18. Heid CA, Stevens J, Livak KJ, et al. Real time quantitative PCR. Genome Res 1990,0.980–94.
19. Furet JP, Firmesse O, le Gourmelon M, et al. Comparative assessment of human and farm animal faecal microbiota using real-time quantitative PCR. FEMS Microbiol Ecol 2009;68:351–62.
20. Hartman AL, Lough DM, Barupal DK, et al. Human gut microbiome adopts an alternative state following small bowel transplantation. Proc Natl Acad Sci U S A 2009;106:17187–92.
21. Guschin DY, Mobarry BK, Proudnikov D, et al. Oligonucleotide microchips as genosensors for determinative and environmental studies in microbiology. Appl Environ Microbiol 1997;63:2397–402.
22. Rajilic-Stojanovic M, Heilig HG, Molenaar D, et al. Development and application of the human intestinal tract chip, a phylogenetic microarray: analysis of universally conserved phylotypes in the abundant microbiota of young and elderly adults. Environ Microbiol 2009;11:1736–51.

23. Kuczynski J, Lauber CL, Walters WA, et al. Experimental and analytical tools for studying the human microbiome. Nat Rev Genet 2011;13:47–58.

24. Liu Z, Lozupone C, Hamady M, et al. Short pyrosequencing reads suffice for accurate microbial community analysis. Nucleic Acids Res 2007;35:e120.

25. Frank DN, Pace NR. Gastrointestinal microbiology enters the metagenomics era. Curr Opin Gastroenterol 2008;24:4–10.

26. Palmer C, Bik EM, DiGiulio DB, et al. Development of the human infant intestinal microbiota. PLoS Biol 2007;5:e177.

27. Liu Z, DeSantis TZ, Andersen GL, et al. Accurate taxonomy assignments from 16S rRNA sequences produced by highly parallel pyrosequencers. Nucleic Acids Res 2008;36:e120.

28. Caporaso JG, Kuczynski J, Stombaugh J, et al. QIIME allows analysis of high-throughput community sequencing data. Nat Methods 2010;7:335–6.

29. Schloss PD, Westcott SL, Ryabin T, et al. Introducing mothur: open-source, platform-independent, community-supported software for describing and comparing microbial communities. Appl Environ Microbiol 2009;75:7537–41.

30. Turnbaugh PJ, Hamady M, Yatsunenko T, et al. A core gut microbiome in obese and lean twins. Nature 2009;457:480–4.

31. Kurokawa K, Itoh T, Kuwahara T, et al. Comparative metagenomics revealed commonly enriched gene sets in human gut microbiomes. DNA Res 2007;14: 169–81.

32. Benson DA, Karsch-Mizrachi I, Clark K, et al. GenBank. Nucleic Acids Res 2012; 40:D48–53.

33. Kanehisa M, Goto S. KEGG: Kyoto encyclopedia of genes and genomes. Nucleic Acids Res 2000;28:27–30.

34. Grigoriev IV, Nordberg H, Shabalov I, et al. The genome portal of the department of energy joint genome institute. Nucleic Acids Res 2012;40:D26–32.

35. Arumugam M, Harrington ED, Foerstner KU, et al. SmashCommunity: a metagenomic annotation and analysis tool. Bioinformatics 2010;26:2977–8.

36. Kosakovsky Pond S, Wadhawan S, Chiaromonte F, et al. Windshield splatter analysis with the Galaxy metagenomic pipeline. Genome Res 2009;19:2144–53.

37. Qin J, Li R, Raes J, et al. A human gut microbial gene catalogue established by metagenomic sequencing. Nature 2010;464:59–65.

38. Moran MA. Metatranscriptomics: eavesdropping on complex microbial communities. Microbe 2009;4:329–35.

39. Stewart FJ, Ottesen EA, DeLong EF. Development and quantitative analyses of a universal rRNA-subtraction protocol for microbial metatranscriptomics. ISME J 2010;4:896–907.

40. Tannock GW, Lawley B, Munro K, et al. Comprehensive analysis of the bacterial content of stool from patients with chronic pouchitis, normal pouches, or familial adenomatous polyposis pouches. Inflamm Bowel Dis 2012;18:925–34.

41. Madden MV, McIntyre AS, Nicholls RJ. Double-blind crossover trial of metronidazole versus placebo in chronic unremitting pouchitis. Dig Dis Sci 1994;39: 1193–6.

A Commentary on the Safety of Probiotics

Fergus Shanahan, MD

KEYWORDS

• Commensals • Microbiota • Lactobacillus • Bifidobacterium

KEY POINTS

- Probiotics have a long record of safety, which relates primarily to lactobacilli and bifido-bacteria. Experience with other forms of probiotics is more limited.
- There is no such thing as zero risk, particularly in the context of certain forms of host susceptibility.
- There is poor public understanding of the concept of risk in general and risk/benefit analysis in particular.
- Uncertainty persists regarding the potential for transfer of antibiotic resistance with probiotics, but the risk seems to be low with currently available probiotic products.
- As with other forms of therapeutics, the safety of probiotics should be considered on a strain-by-strain basis.

INTRODUCTION

"Medicine used to be simple, ineffective and relatively safe. Now it is complex, effective and potentially dangerous"

—*Cyril Chantler, Lancet 1999*[1]

Some would contest the aforementioned statement claiming that medical remedies have been dangerous since the age of Hippocrates and before. The statement reflects the risks and benefits of modern drugs, such as immunomodulatory biologic agents, but does not adequately describe all forms of modern medicine and, in particular, the low risk with modest benefit offered by most probiotics currently in use. Any discussion of probiotic safety would be misleading were it not to acknowledge the remarkably low rate of adverse events recorded with probiotic consumption, either as specific products in the context of controlled trials or as constituents in fermented

FS is funded, in part, by Science Foundation Ireland in the form of a research center grant, the *Alimentary Pharmabiotic Center*. FS has consulted for and/or received research grants from Alimentary Health Ltd and GlaxoSmithKline Ltd. The content of this article was neither influenced nor constrained by these facts.
Department of Medicine, Alimentary Pharmabiotic Centre, University College Cork, National University of Ireland, Cork, Ireland
E-mail address: F.Shanahan@ucc.ie

Gastroenterol Clin N Am 41 (2012) 869–876
http://dx.doi.org/10.1016/j.gtc.2012.08.006
0889-8553/12/$ – see front matter © 2012 Elsevier Inc. All rights reserved.

food products, over a long history of widespread use. However, there are important caveats regarding probiotic safety that need emphasis.

First, the safety record of probiotic strains in current use does not necessarily apply to new strains in development and each needs assessment on a case-by-case basis. Second, probiotic strains are highly varied without a uniform mechanism of action and, therefore, unlikely to have the same adverse effects in all situations. Third, there is no such thing as zero risk, whether for drugs, probiotics, or even therapeutic nihilism. Fourth, there is poor public understanding of risk in general and risk/benefit analysis in particular, which needs to be addressed. Fifth, because some probiotic products are marketed to those seeking alternative medicine in health-food stores or are available from sources under dubious regulatory constraints, the quality of the product in terms of potential contaminants may be more important than concerns regarding the specific properties of the probiotic constituent. Finally, although probiotics have commonly been selected from the nonpathogenic components of the commensal microbiota and generally regarded as safe, the relationship between commensals and pathogens is not one of mutual opposites, but rather they are at different positions on a spectrum of low to high pathogenic potential.

Probiotics are usually defined as "live microorganisms, which when administered in adequate amounts confer a health benefit on the host."[2] The limitations of the restrictive nature of this definition have been commented on elsewhere because it excludes dead organisms, probiotic fragments, and metabolites, such as bioactive polysaccharides, nucleotides, and proteins.[3] Like the fate of the original definition of antibiotics, which excluded sulphonamides and synthetic antimicrobials, the definition of probiotics may have outlived its usefulness and is likely to undergo refinements that will be informed by science. At present, yeast (*Saccharomyces cervisiae*) and bacteria comply with the current definition of probiotics with the latter including species of *Lactobacillus*, *Streptococcus*, *Enterococcus*, *Bifidobacterium*, *Propionibacterium*, *Bacillus*, and *Escherichia coli*. In addition, the organisms may be either naturally occurring or genetically modified. This degree of heterogeneity underscores the problem of using a collective generic name. In the same way that the safety and efficacy of drugs would never be addressed in collective, generic terms, so probiotic bacteria need consideration individually on a case-by-case basis, particularly those still in development.

WHEN FRIENDLY BACTERIA BEHAVE POORLY

Because consumption of a probiotic represents, in essence, an intention to mimic, supplement, or otherwise harness the commensal microbiota, the distinction between commensals and pathogens becomes critical. Organisms with a propensity to cross biologic boundaries, like the mucosal barrier, are obviously pathogens; but the distinction from commensals is not always readily evident, particularly when the host has a particular vulnerability, such as an acquired barrier defect or a genetic susceptibility. How does the host distinguish pathogens from commensals or consumed probiotics? This process is complex and cannot be based solely on the recognition of microbe-associated molecular patterns because the patterns involved in the recognition of pathogens are also expressed by nonpathogens, including probiotics.[4]

The problem is solved for some commensals by the production of symbiosis-associated molecular patterns. This point is exemplified by *Bacteroides fragilis*, a prominent member of the commensal microbiota, which produces an immunomodulatory polysaccharide that signals through Toll-like receptor 2 on regulatory T cells within the host to suppress T_H17 effectors, thereby avoiding an adverse immune response.[5] The degree to which this mechanism is deployed by other commensals/probiotics is unclear, but the host has a backup surveillance system for the detection of danger signals from the microbiota and for modifying the composition of the microenvironment. This detection is achieved by the inflammasomes, which are intracellular multi-protein complexes that sense exogenous and endogenous stress or damage. Experimental defects in inflammasome function have shown their importance within the epithelium and mucosal phagocytes, not only in detecting pathogenic components within the microbiota but also in initiating a cascade of immunologic responses to restore compositional equilibrium within the microbiota.[6,7]

Of course, some organisms may, depending on the context and/or depending on the host susceptibility, behave either as a commensal or as a pathogen. The clearest example of commensals in the wrong place at the wrong time is that of the baby born too soon, born before maturation of the mucosal and blood-brain barriers, and before full development of immunity. In this setting, colonization with what would otherwise be considered harmless commensals poses a threat. The case for using probiotics in premature infants has been well made, albeit still controversial.[8–12] Regardless, the use of probiotics in premature infants is not without risk and should be considered as an attempt to substitute organisms of low pathogenic risk for those that may represent greater risk to the vulnerable neonate.

The importance of context in relation to risk and benefit is also illustrated by the case of *Helicobacter pylori*. Many clinicians have adopted the unidimensional view that the only good *H. pylori* is a dead *H. pylori*, but the outcome of the host-helicobacter interaction may be favorable, unfavorable, or both for the host, depending on the bacterial strain and on a variety of factors, including the age and susceptibility of the host.[13–15] The organism is usually acquired in childhood but only after a variable period of apparent health causes peptic ulceration in adulthood in a minority of those infected. At a later age, the organism may cause gastric cancer. The potential benefits from the same organism also depend on the age of the host. In early life, *H pylori* may protect against asthma and infections; but later, it protects against reflux-associated complications, such as metaplasia and neoplasia at the gastroesophageal junction.

JUST THE FACTS…

The safety record of probiotics has been the subject of several thoughtful systematic reviews over the past decade.[16–22] The overwhelming consensus has been one of relative, but not zero, safety. Well-documented cases of sepsis presumed or proven to be linked with lactobacilli and bifidobacteria have been reported but are rare.[23,24] Such organisms transmigrate across the mucosal barrier less readily than other commensals, but this feature may not apply to all probiotics in the future, particularly those from different genera.[20,25] It must be emphasized that most experience with probiotics has been with lactobacilli and bifidobacteria; the safety record with other forms of probiotic, such as enterococci, may differ and needs more measured and qualified confidence.[22] In addition, although concern has been expressed about the risk of probiotics in vulnerable groups, such as the immunosuppressed or those with an abnormal mucosal barrier, the record to date is encouraging.[21,23,26–28] Continual vigilance for unanticipated adverse effects is warranted. The more striking aspects of the safety record are outlined in **Box 1**.

More recently, the US Agency for Health care Research and Quality commissioned the Southern California Evidence-Based Practice Center, based at RAND, to conduct a systematic review of the safety of probiotics.[29] The review was sponsored by the National Institutes of Health and by the Food and Drug Administration and was based on an analysis of trials using probiotics to reduce risk and prevent or treat disease.

Box 1
Overview of human safety record associated with probiotic consumption

Major safety considerations

Approximately a century of experience

Lactobacillus infection estimated at 1 per 10^7 in France

Risk of lactobacillemia less than 1 per 10^6

No increase in Finland with increased consumption of *L rhamnosus* GG

Impressive safety record in immunocompromised patients (eg, human immunodeficiency virus, premature infants, the elderly, inflammatory bowel disease)

Low (not zero) opportunistic pathogenicity

Sparse safety record of nonlactobacillus and nonbfidobacterial strains

Particular hygienic precautions are required for patients with a central venous catheter and some advise avoidance of S. boulardii in these patients. Others advise avoidance of probiotics in patients with synthetic cardiac valve replacement

Data from Sanders ME, Akkermans LM, Haller D, et al. Safety assessment of probiotics for human use. Gut Microbes 2010;1:164–85.

The investigators concluded that the available evidence in randomized controlled trials does not indicate an increased risk but cautioned that rare adverse events are difficult to assess and that the available literature is not well suited to answer specific questions on safety. A commentary on the report has been offered by Wallace and MacKay[30] who argue that the safety record of probiotics should be judged not by controlled trials alone but on the totality of the evidence, including a long history of safe use in healthy populations in the form of fermented food products along with animal experiments, all of which point toward safety.[30]

ANTIBIOTIC RESISTANCE AND TRANSFER

Resistance to antibiotics and, more importantly, the potential transfer of antibiotic resistance from fed probiotics to the commensal microbiota in vivo is an important ongoing concern and underscores the importance of whole-genome sequencing of candidate probiotic strains. This subject has been discussed in detail elsewhere. Although it remains a valid concern,[20,21] there is little evidence that it is a significant problem in vivo with currently available probiotic products, although it seems to be a greater risk with enterococci than with lactobacilli and bifidobacteria.[21] A high degree of genetic stability has been associated with lactobacillus and bifidobacterium strains used in commercial probiotics, but the risk of transfer of antibiotic resistance determinants under different conditions of production and storage in vivo needs continual assessment and vigilance.

DESIGNER TURBO PROBIOTICS

Strictly speaking, genetically engineered organisms may comply with the current definition of a probiotic but need special consideration on a case-by-case basis and are likely to be viewed as pharmaceuticals from a regulatory perspective. Safety issues involve not only the carrier organism but also the recombinant product engineered for production by the organism. Furthermore, the issue of safety does not stop at the level of the individual consumer; public health concerns regarding the containment of the genetically altered strain from the wider environment, after excretion, need additional attention.

Insertion of the therapeutic transgene into the bacterial *thy A* locus, which codes for thymidylate synthase, renders the organism dependent on thymine or thymidine in the local microenvironment, thereby limiting its viability after excretion. If the engineered organism reacquires the *thy A* gene, the transgene is eliminated from the bacterial genome. The safety and efficacy of this strategy has been explored experimentally with the food-grade organism, *Lactococcus lactis,* engineered to express, inter alia, interleukin 10, trefoil factor, and anti–tumor necrosis factor nanobodies.[31–33]

An alternative approach has been to use an anaerobic commensal, *Bacteroides ovatus*, engineered to produce either keratinocyte growth factor or transforming growth factor-beta under the control of dietary xylan, with efficacy in experimental inflammatory bowel disease.[34,35] Containment and biosafety are assured by this clever strategy, in part, by the anaerobic dependency of the organism and by the dietary dependency of its engineered product.

TALES OF THE UNEXPECTED
Probiotics and Pancreatitis

One of the more striking adverse outcomes linked with probiotic consumption was a report of a higher-than-expected mortality rate in patients receiving a multispecies probiotic preparation in the context of a double-blind placebo-controlled trial of prophylaxis in predicted severe acute pancreatitis (PROPATRIA study).[36] The increased mortality in the probiotic limb was attributed to bowel ischemia. Remarkably, the editors of the journal in which the trial was published subsequently issued an expression of concern about the study based on an investigation by Dutch regulatory authorities.[37] The investigation detected shortcomings in the design and conduct of the trial. In correspondence with the journal, the authors of the original report made the quite reasonable point that best practices of the time were followed for the trial.[38] In other correspondence, the conclusions of the original trial report were challenged and rebutted. One group of correspondents claimed that the microbial product used in the trial did not precisely match the current definition of a probiotic and, therefore, the conclusion did not pertain to probiotics.[39] The latter argument is unconvincing, circular, and illustrates the folly of clinging to outdated definitions and rhetoric to absolve probiotics of risk. Regardless of the flaws in the design, execution, or interpretation of the PROPATRIA trial, sufficient concern has been raised to justify caution with the use of certain types of probiotics in acutely ill patients. In the future, the potential benefits should outweigh the theoretical risks and these should be evaluated carefully.

Probiotics and Obesity

A speculative editorial raised a concern regarding a possible link between probiotic usage and obesity. This concern was based entirely on circumstantial evidence, such as the use of probiotics as growth promoters in the farming industry.[40] The logic and evidence supporting this contention have been contested by others, with the counterargument that probiotics are actually used to promote lean body mass and not adiposity in livestock.[41,42] In the latter context, probiotics might actually serve an untapped role in combating the sarcopenia that may arise in the elderly or in patients with cancer. A comparative meta-analysis of different lactobacillus species on weight gain in humans and animals claimed that different lactobacillus species vary in their apparent effects on weight change, which are host specific.[43]

WHAT IS ON THE LABEL? WHAT IS REALLY IN IT?

Safety assessments of probiotic products should not be limited to consideration of the active probiotic constituent; the potential for microbial contaminants is probably a greater concern along with misleading or inaccurate labeling. Anyone perusing the shelves of convenience stores, pharmacies, and health-food outlets in the United States will have no difficulty finding over-the-counter probiotic products emblazoned with dramatic claims on their labels, few, if any, of which have been scientifically confirmed. Buyers can, however, exercise discretion because misleading labels and claims are far less likely when the product is from a long-established and reputable company.

Although in some surveys the quality control of certain probiotics has fared well,[44] several retail products have been found to contain microbes that were not identified on the label.[45–48] This circumstance is more likely to be caused by dubious quality control rather than intentional deception of the customer. The potential for microbial contamination in the production process is substantial, and this underscores again the importance of choosing a reputable supplier. It also means that safety assessments are unreliable if the producer is unaware of the precise contents and quantities thereof in their products. Potential hazards are not limited to microbiologic components and include the risk of allergies to milk and other allergens in probiotic products, which should be specified on the label.[49]

SUMMARY

Probiotics have a long record of safety. However, zero risk does not exist. Vigilance is required for unexpected adverse effects, particularly as new strains emerge and as probiotic use becomes more widespread and may be used in hosts with genetic or acquired susceptibilities. In that respect, it is important to acknowledge that the distinction between a commensal or probiotic and a pathogen is often a matter of context. Of continuing importance is the uncertainty surrounding antibiotic resistance transfer. Probiotic quality control may be even more important than assessment of the properties of the probiotic constituent itself. However, discussing probiotics in collective or generic terms is like speaking of tablets or pills without addressing the specific pharmaceutical content of the pill and the indication for which it is used. Thus, the time is long past when probiotics should be considered in specific terms on a strain-by-strain basis.

REFERENCES

1. Chantler C. The role and education of doctors in the delivery of health care. Lancet 1999;353:1178–81.
2. FAO/WHO Health and nutritional properties of probiotics in food including powder milk with live lactic acid bacteria. 2001. Available at: http://www.who.int/foodsafety/publications/fs_management/en/probiotics.pdf. Accessed June 4, 2012.
3. Shanahan F, Stanton C, Ross P, et al. Pharmabiotics: bioactives from mining host-microbe-dietary interactions. Functional Food Rev 2009;1:20–5.
4. Lebeer S, Vanderleyden J, De Keersmaecker SC. Host interactions of probiotic bacterial surface molecules: comparison with commensals and pathogens. Nat Rev Microbiol 2010;8:171–84.
5. Round JL, Lee SM, Li J, et al. The Toll-like receptor 2 pathway establishes colonization by a commensal of the human microbiota. Science 2011;332:974–7.
6. Elinav E, Strowig T, Kau AL, et al. NLRP6 inflammasome regulates colonic microbial ecology and risk for colitis. Cell 2011;145:1–13.

7. Franchi L, Kamada N, Namamura Y, et al. NLRC4-driven production on IL-1β discriminates between pathogenic and commensal bacteria and promotes host intestinal disease. Nat Immunol 2012;13:449–56.

8. Shanahan F. Probiotics in perspective. Gastroenterology 2010;139:1808–12.

9. Deshpande G, Rao S, Patole S, et al. Updated meta-analysis of probiotics for preventing necrotizing enterocolitis in preterm neonates. Pediatrics 2010;125:921–30.

10. Tarnow-Mordi WO, Wilkinson D, Trivedi A, et al. Probiotics reduce all-cause mortality and necrotizing enterocolitis: it is time to change practice. Pediatrics 2010;125:1068–70.

11. Soll RF. Probiotics: are we ready for routine use? Pediatrics 2010;125:1071–2.

12. Mihatsch WA, Braegger CP, Decsi T, et al. Critical systematic review of the level of evidence for routine use of probiotics for reduction of mortality and prevention of necrotizing enterocolitis and sepsis in preterm infants. Clin Nutr 2012;31:6–15.

13. Blaser MJ. Heterogeneity of Helicobacter pylori. Eur J Gastroenterol Hepatol 2012;9(Suppl 1):S3–6 [discussion: S6–7].

14. Blaser MJ. Helicobacter pylori and esophageal disease: wake-up call? Gastroenterology 2010;139:1819–22.

15. Blaser MJ, Falkow S. What are the consequences of the disappearing human microbiota? Nat Rev Microbiol 2009;7:887–94.

16. Boyle RJ, Robins-Browne RM, Tang ML. Probiotic use in clinical medicine: what are the risks? Am J Clin Nutr 2006;83:1256–64.

17. Whelan K, Myers CE. Safety of probiotics in patients receiving nutritional support: a systematic review of case reports, randomised controlled trials, and nonrandomised trials. Am J Clin Nutr 2010;91:687–703.

18. Bernardeau M, Vernoux JP, Henri-Dubernet S, et al. Safety assessment of dairy microorganisms: the Lactobacillus genus. Int J Food Microbiol 2008;126:278–85.

19. Snydman DR. The safety of probiotics. Clin Infect Dis 2008;46:S104–11.

20. Abe F, Muto M, Yaeshima T, et al. Safety evaluation of probiotic bifidobacteria by analysis of mucin degradation activity and translocation ability. Anaerobe 2010;16:131–6.

21. Sanders ME, Akkermans LM, Haller D, et al. Safety assessment of probiotics for human use. Gut Microbes 2010;1:164–85.

22. Franz CM, Huch M, Abriouel H, et al. Enterococci as probiotics and their implications in food safety. Int J Food Microbiol 2011;151:125–40.

23. Conen A, Zimmerer S, Frei R, et al. A pain in the neck: probiotics for ulcerative colitis. Ann Intern Med 2009;151:U9S–7.

24. Ohishi A, Takahashi S, Ito Y, et al. Bifidobacterium septicaemia associated with postoperative probiotic therapy in a neonate with omphalocele. J Pediatr 2010;156:679–81.

25. Lapthorne S, MacSharry J, Scully P, et al. Differential M cell gene expression in response to gut commensals. Immunology 2012;136:312–24.

26. Wagner RD, Balish E. Potential hazards of probiotic bacteria for immunodeficient patients. Bull Inst Pasteur 1998;96:165–70.

27. Hedin C, Whelan K, Lindsay JO. Evidence for the use of probiotics and prebiotics in inflammatory bowel disease: a review of clinical trials. Proc Nutr Soc 2007;66:307–15.

28. Steed H, Macfarlane GT, Macfaralne S. Prebiotics, synbiotics and inflammatory bowel disease. Mol Nutr Food Res 2008;52:898–905.

29. Hempel S, Newberry S, Ruelaz A, et al. Safety of probiotics to reduce risk and prevent or treat disease. Evidence-based practice centre under contract

no. 11-E007. Rockville (MD): Agency for Healthcare Research and Quality; 2011. Available at: www.ahrq.gov/clinic/tp/probiotictp.htm. Accessed June 1, 2012.

30. Wallace TC, MacKay D. The safety of probiotics: considerations following the 2011 U.S. Agency for Health Research and Quality report. J Nutr 2011;141: 1923–4.

31. Steidler L, Hans W, Schotte L, et al. Treatment of murine colitis by Lactococcus lactis secreting interleukin-10. Science 2000;289:1352–5.

32. Braat H, Rottiers P, Hommes DW, et al. A phase I trial with transgenic bacteria expressing interleukin-10 in Crohn's disease. Clin Gastroenterol Hepatol 2006; 4:754–9.

33. Vandenbroucke K, de Haard H, Beirnaert E, et al. Orally administered L. lactis secreting an anti-TNF Nanobody demonstrate efficacy in chronic colitis. Mucosal Immunol 2009;3:49–56.

34. Hamady ZZ, Scott N, Farrar MD, et al. Xylan-regulated delivery of human keratinocyte growth factor-2 to the inflamed colon by the human anaerobic commensal bacterium Bacteroides ovatus. Gut 2010;59:461–9.

35. Hamady ZZ, Scott N, Farrar MD, et al. Treatment of colitis with a commensal gut bacterium engineered to secrete human TGF-β1 under the control of dietary xylan 1. Inflamm Bowel Dis 2011;17:1925–35.

36. Besselink MG, Santvoort HC, Buskens E, et al. Probiotic prophylaxis in predicted severe acute pancreatitis: a randomised, double-blind, placebo-controlled trial. Lancet 2008;371:651–9.

37. The Editors of the Lancet Expression of concern – Probiotic prophylaxis in predicted severe acute pancreatitis: a randomised, double-blind, placebo-controlled trial. Lancet 2010;375:875–6.

38. Gooszen HG, on behalf of the Dutch pancreatitis study group. The PROPATRIA trial: best practices at the time were followed. Lancet 2010;375:1249–50.

39. Reid G, Gibson G, Sanders ME, et al. Probiotic prophylaxis in predicted acute severe pancreatitis. Lancet 2008;372:112–3.

40. Raoult D. Probiotics and obesity: a link? Nat Rev Microbiol 2009;7:616.

41. Ehrlich SD. Probiotics – little evidence for a link to obesity. Nat Rev Microbiol 2009;7:901.

42. Delzenne N, Reid G. No causal link between obesity and probiotics. Nat Rev Microbiol 2009;7:901.

43. Million M, Angelakis E, Paul M, et al. Comparative meta-analysis of the effect of Lactobacillus species on weight gain in humans and animals. Microb Pathog 2012;53(2):100–8.

44. Vanhee LM, Goemé F, Nelis HJ, et al. Quality control of fifteen probiotic products containing Saccharomyces boulardii. J Appl Microbiol 2010;109:1745–52.

45. Masco L, Huys G, De Brandt E, et al. Culture-dependent and culture-independent qualitative analysis of probiotic products claimed to contain bifidobacteria. Int J Food Microbiol 2005;102:221–30.

46. Temmerman R, Scheirlinck I, Huys G, et al. Culture-independent analysis of probiotic products by denaturing gradient gel electrophoresis. Appl Environ Microbiol 2003;69:220–6.

47. Coeuret V, Gueguen M, Vernoux JP. Numbers and strains of lactobacilli in some probiotic products. Int J Food Microbiol 2004;97:147–56.

48. Weese JS. Evaluation of deficiencies in labeling of commercial probiotics. Can Vet J 2003;44:982–3.

49. Moneret-Vautrin DA, Morisset M, Cordebar V, et al. Probiotics may be unsafe in infants allergic to cow's milk. Allergy 2006;61:507–8.

Index

Note: Page numbers of article titles are in **boldface** type.

A

Adenosine AMP-AMP activation, in obesity, 846
Allergic disease, **747–762**
 challenges of, 748–749, 758
 hygiene hypothesis and, 747–748
 intestinal microbiota status and, 722–723, 749–752
 maternal exposure to animals and, 719–720
 probiotics for, 753–758
  challenges in, 758
  in established disease, 755, 758
  preventative, 754–757
Amniotic fluid, intestinal microbiota and, 719–720
Amplicon sequencing, 863
Anorexia nervosa, probiotics for, 793
Antibiotics
 diarrhea associated with, **763–779**
  causes of, 764
  Clostridium difficile colitis with, 769–776
  definition of, 763–764
  probiotics for
   Helicobacter pylori therapy with, 768
   mechanisms of action of, 765
   preventive, 764–765, 767–769
   single-strain, 765–766
 intestinal microbiota composition and, 722
 resistance to, transfer to commensals, 872
Asthma, intestinal microbiota composition and, 722–723
Atopic disease. *See* Allergic disease.
Autism, probiotics for, 794–795

B

Bacteroides, in infant intestinal microbiota, 732
Bacteroides fragilis, as commensal, 870–871
Baker hypothesis, for adult disease development, 719
BIFCO, for ulcerative colitis, 827
Bifidobacterium
 for allergic disease, 755–757
 for antibiotic-associated diarrhea, 767
 for Crohn disease, 833–834, 836
 for irritable bowel syndrome, 808, 810
 for obesity, 847, 849–850

Gastroenterol Clin N Am 41 (2012) 877–884
http://dx.doi.org/10.1016/S0889-8553(12)00113-6
0889-8553/12/$ – see front matter © 2012 Elsevier Inc. All rights reserved.

United States Postal Service

Statement of Ownership, Management, and Circulation
(All Periodicals Publications Except Requestor Publications)

1. Publication Title	2. Publication Number	3. Filing Date
Gastroenterology Clinics of North America	0 0 0 - 2 7 7 9	9/14/12

4. Issue Frequency	5. Number of Issues Published Annually	6. Annual Subscription Price
Mar, Jun, Sep, Dec	4	$305.00

7. Complete Mailing Address of Known Office of Publication (*Not printer*) (*Street, city, county, state, and ZIP+4®*)

Elsevier Inc.
360 Park Avenue South
New York, NY 10010-1710

Contact Person
Stephen R. Bushing
Telephone (*Include area code*)
215-239-3688

8. Complete Mailing Address of Headquarters or General Business Office of Publisher (*Not printer*)

Elsevier Inc., 360 Park Avenue South, New York, NY 10010-1710

9. Full Names and Complete Mailing Addresses of Publisher, Editor, and Managing Editor (*Do not leave blank*)

Publisher (*Name and complete mailing address*)

Kim Murphy, Elsevier, Inc., 1600 John F. Kennedy Blvd. Suite 1800, Philadelphia, PA 19103-2899

Editor (*Name and complete mailing address*)

Kerry Holland, Elsevier, Inc., 1600 John F. Kennedy Blvd. Suite 1800, Philadelphia, PA 19103-2899

Managing Editor (*Name and complete mailing address*)

Sarah Barth, Elsevier, Inc., 1600 John F. Kennedy Blvd. Suite 1800, Philadelphia, PA 19103-2899

10. Owner (*Do not leave blank. If the publication is owned by a corporation, give the name and address of the corporation immediately followed by the names and addresses of all stockholders owning or holding 1 percent or more of the total amount of stock. If not owned by a corporation, give the names and addresses of the individual owners. If owned by a partnership or other unincorporated firm, give its name and address as well as those of each individual owner. If the publication is published by a nonprofit organization, give its name and address.*)

Full Name	Complete Mailing Address
Wholly owned subsidiary of	1600 John F. Kennedy Blvd., Ste. 1800
Reed/Elsevier, US holdings	Philadelphia, PA 19103-2899

11. Known Bondholders, Mortgagees, and Other Security Holders Owning or Holding 1 Percent or More of Total Amount of Bonds, Mortgages, or Other Securities. If none, check box ☑ None

Full Name	Complete Mailing Address
N/A	

12. Tax Status (*For completion by nonprofit organizations authorized to mail at nonprofit rates*) (*Check one*)
The purpose, function, and nonprofit status of this organization and the exempt status for federal income tax purposes:
☐ Has Not Changed During Preceding 12 Months
☐ Has Changed During Preceding 12 Months (*Publisher must submit explanation of change with this statement*)

PS Form 3526, September 2007 (Page 1 of 3 (Instructions Page 3)) PSN 7530-01-000-9931 PRIVACY NOTICE: See our Privacy policy in www.usps.com

---

13. Publication Title	14. Issue Date for Circulation Data Below
Gastroenterology Clinics of North America	September 2012

15. Extent and Nature of Circulation			Average No. Copies Each Issue During Preceding 12 Months	No. Copies of Single Issue Published Nearest to Filing Date
a. Total Number of Copies (*Net press run*)			996	995
b. Paid Circulation (By Mail and Outside the Mail)	(1)	Mailed Outside-County Paid Subscriptions Stated on PS Form 3541. (*Include paid distribution above nominal rate, advertiser's proof copies, and exchange copies*)	393	355
	(2)	Mailed In-County Paid Subscriptions Stated on PS Form 3541 (*Include paid distribution above nominal rate, advertiser's proof copies, and exchange copies*)		
	(3)	Paid Distribution Outside the Mails Including Sales Through Dealers and Carriers, Street Vendors, Counter Sales, and Other Paid Distribution Outside USPS®	259	299
	(4)	Paid Distribution by Other Classes Mailed Through the USPS (e.g. First-Class Mail®)		
c. Total Paid Distribution (Sum of 15b (1), (2), (3), and (4))		▲	652	654
d. Free or Nominal Rate Distribution (By Mail and Outside the Mail)	(1)	Free or Nominal Rate Outside-County Copies Included on PS Form 3541	93	101
	(2)	Free or Nominal Rate In-County Copies Included on PS Form 3541		
	(3)	Free or Nominal Rate Copies Mailed at Other Classes Through the USPS (e.g. First-Class Mail)		
	(4)	Free or Nominal Rate Distribution Outside the Mail (Carriers or other means)		
e. Total Free or Nominal Rate Distribution (Sum of 15d (1), (2), (3) and (4))		▲	93	101
f. Total Distribution (Sum of 15c and 15e)		▲	745	755
g. Copies not Distributed (See instructions to publishers #4 (page #3))		▲	251	240
h. Total (Sum of 15f and g)		▲	996	995
i. Percent Paid (15c divided by 15f times 100)			87.52%	86.62%

16. Publication of Statement of Ownership
If the publication is a general publication, publication of this statement is required. Will be printed in the **December 2012** issue of this publication. ☐ Publication not required

17. Signature and Title of Editor, Publisher, Business Manager, or Owner

Stephen R. Bushing – Inventory Distribution Coordinator

Date
September 14, 2012

I certify that all information furnished on this form is true and complete. I understand that anyone who furnishes false or misleading information on this form or who omits material or information requested on the form may be subject to criminal sanctions (including fines and imprisonment) and/or civil sanctions (including civil penalties).

PS Form 3526, September 2007 (Page 2 of 3)

Moving?

Make sure your subscription moves with you!

To notify us of your new address, find your **Clinics Account Number** (located on your mailing label above your name), and contact customer service at:

Email: journalscustomerservice-usa@elsevier.com

800-654-2452 (subscribers in the U.S. & Canada)
314-447-8871 (subscribers outside of the U.S. & Canada)

Fax number: 314-447-8029

Elsevier Health Sciences Division
Subscription Customer Service
3251 Riverport Lane
Maryland Heights, MO 63043

*To ensure uninterrupted delivery of your subscription, please notify us at least 4 weeks in advance of move.

Printed and bound by CPI Group (UK) Ltd, Croydon, CR0 4YY

03/10/2024

01040461-0016